I0407492

The Anti-Aging Secret

A Natural Essential Oils Guide to Staying Young

by Ann Sullivan

Published in USA by:

Ann Sullivan
217 N. Seacrest Blvd #9
Boynton Beach
FL 33425

© Copyright 2015

ISBN-13: ISBN-13: 978-1544739076
ISBN-10: ISBN-10: 1544739079

ALL RIGHTS RESERVED. No part of this publication may be reproduced or transmitted in any form whatsoever, electronic, or mechanical, including photocopying, recording, or by any informational storage or retrieval system without express written, dated and signed permission from the author.

Introduction

What are essential oils, and how might they be used for therapeutic purposes?

Essential oils are ultra-potent oils, extracted from plants and flowers that have been utilized in medicine for centuries. Presently, they are more commonly used to supplement pharmaceutical medication, but they can also be an effective alternative to pharmaceuticals in the event that you don't have access to them. Before you dismiss essential oils as a means to support the body's natural defenses against injuries and illness, take a look at the historical evidence of the oils' medicinal competence in practice. Your average age-old medical text will demonstrate that essential oils, herbs, and plenty of other natural ingredients have, for thousands of years, successfully enhanced immune function to meet and defeat any number of ailments and injuries. Though traditional medicine is considered "alternative" now, it was once the gold standard and, quite frankly, it still should be, as these natural historic remedies can fortify the body's defenses against everything from simple maladies, like headaches, cuts, and bruises, to serious diseases.

Essential oils are deemed "essential," because the oils are composed of the "essence" of the plant. The difference between essential oils and other oils – like olive oil or vegetable oil, for instance – is that essential oils have high volatility and reduced fixation, which results in faster evaporation, enabling their popular use in aromatherapy. Even at high temperatures, olive and vegetable oils don't evaporate.

You probably don't realize that you already use essential oils every day. They're in perfumes, shampoos, soaps, ointments...they're even used in furniture polish. Why are they found in so many aromatic products? Well, basically, because essential oils are super concentrated aromatic liquids, so their scent is remarkably strong. Let's put this into perspective: to steam tea, you use a few leaves of Peppermint or Juniper; to produce a single ounce of essential oil, five whole *pounds* of Peppermint or Juniper leaves are required. Some sources claim that to produce twelve pounds of essential oil would necessitate an acre of Peppermint. So, unlike vegetable oil, you do not find concentrated therapeutic-grade essential oils sold in bulk; instead the oils are often sold in easily carried small, dark bottles.

Now that we have an idea of what essential oils are, let's discuss how can they help with aging? Although we are not getting any younger, and aging is a natural process, our habits can impact the rate and severity at which we age. There is no elixir of youth; being the fittest and healthiest that you can be, while also taking preventative measures to support your skin and general health is the closest humans can get to fighting against aging. This takes work, consistency, determination, drive, and commitment. Just as with anything that's challenging in life, the effort is worth it if you want to age gracefully.

Unlike your average synthetic anti-aging potions, essential oils are all natural. In regards to therapeutic grade essential oils, there are no added colors, flavors, or preservatives. As previously mentioned, oils are extracted directly from the plant source from which they are derived and so no caffeine or added sugars are injected into these oils to make them "work." The inherent synergy of their chemical components produce supportive properties, including antibacterial, antiviral, antifungal, antiseptic, and antioxidant applications to name just a few.

Essential oils won't make you Benjamin Button, but they can be used to significantly improve those skin, bone, muscle, joint, brain, and sensory conditions that often impact our quality of life as we age. Essential oils can also be used to support the physical issues that contribute to premature aging – such as addiction, sun exposure, free radicals, etc.

Citrus oils are particularly beneficial when it comes to aging. Check out this study, available on PubMed, that examines the antioxidant properties of Lemon and Lime essential oils on aging.

Study 1 – Antioxidant Properties

"Peels and edible pulp from three species of citrus including Citrus aurantifolia (varieties pica and sutil) and Citrus x Lemon var. Genova widely cultivated and consumed in Northern Chile (I and II region) were analyzed for phenolic compounds and antioxidant activity for the first time…The antioxidant features together with the high polyphenolic contents can support at least in part, the usage of the peel extracts as nutraceutical supplements, especially to be used as anti-aging products."

The sole purpose of this study was to analyze the antioxidant properties of Lemon and Lime. Antioxidants protect against free radicals and repair their damage. Although our bodies produce their own antioxidants, these often become damaged as we age, so introducing natural substances that are high in antioxidants into our system allows these nutrients and enzymes to assist in chemical reactions which destroy the oxidants or free radicals. The study evaluated the peels and edible pulp of two varieties of Lime and one of Lemon and demonstrated that the peel extracts are moderate antioxidants, with the potential to serve as dietary supplements or anti-aging ingredients.

Reference:
http://www.ncbi.nlm.nih.gov/pubmed/25356563]
http://www.mdpi.com/1420-3049/19/11/17400]

In this book, we'll discuss seVeral areas of aging, including skin health, bone, muscle, and joint health, brain health, and sensory function. We will offer essential oil and other natural protocols to help provide preventative and ongoing support of these issues. In Chapter 5, we'll also offer a number of essential oil blend recipes that address aging issues.

Chapter 1:
Skin Health

Our skin is one of the toughest and most necessary organs of the body. Not only does our protective layer take the brunt force of many external foes, including UV rays, wind, and even our own bad habits, but it balances fluid and electrolytes in the body, it controls body temperature, and the nerve receptors within the skin enable the brain to process pain, touch, and pressure.

Though skin doesn't appear to be very thick, our armor does include seVeral layers, the three primary of which are the epidermis, the dermis, and the subcutaneous layers. The epidermis is the exterior layer; the layer which we see, and is composed of proteins, pigment, and of course skin cells. The dermis is the middle layer, which delivers nutrients to the epidermis, and is composed of oil glands, nerves, blood vessels, and hair follicles. Lastly, the subcutaneous layer is the innermost layer of skin, which provides durability and flexibility in the skin through its support of the collagen and elastin fibers, by providing these fibers connective tissue. This layer is also composed of fat, blood vessels, sweat glands, and hair follicles.

As external factors are increasingly introduced into our environment, such as pollutants and toxins which can invade the body and interfere with its normal functions, there's no better time than now to upgrade our protective armor. We can fortify our skin, so that it's stronger, lasts longer, and looks better, younger, more supple, and fresher through simple upkeep, and by following general protocols when it comes to personal habits, diet, lifestyle, and other factors that influence skin health, like genetics. By making even minor changes, we can ensure that our skin doesn't look 110, when we're only 45.

Anti-aging Skin Care 101: Essential Oils & Preventative Protocols

As mentioned in the introduction, the rate and intensity of skin aging is a combined result of diet, lifestyle, environment, and heredity factors. When we are talking diet and lifestyle, elements of both include smoking and alcohol consumption, as well as the consumption of junk foods and food items that contain artificial flavorings and preservatives. These factors influence the health of the entire body, so it is no surprise that the instability and over activity of the free radicals (oxygen molecules) produced by smoking and other toxins can cause cell damage. In the case of skin cell damage, premature wrinkles occur.

When we are talking environmental factors, elements include the sun and the toxins/pollutants in the air. As with smoking tobacco, air pollutants introduce oxidants into the skin, leading to cell damage and premature wrinkles. Sun damage is one of the largest contributors to prematurely aging skin. The sun's impact on skin now has a specific term: "photo aging." This term characterizes all skin changes induced by constant and long-term UVA and UVB exposure. This exposure can be either natural or synthetic (tanning booths). Let's take a look at how photo aging works.

Ultraviolet rays from the sun cause damage over time to the elastin of the skin. The strength of these fibers are what determine the skin's elasticity, so when they're weakened, the skin sags, stretches, and does not snap back from stretching as easily. The weakening also contributes to easier tearing and bruising of the skin, which makes the healing process from minor cuts and scrapes last a lot longer. Though sun damage may not be altogether visible in your youth, it accumulates over time and can affect the age of your skin in later life.

Although, like the rest of the body, the skin is conditioned to repair itself and return to homeostasis, intensive sun damage cannot be completely repaired, so it's best to take preventative measures when you plan to be out in the sun. This means wearing hats, covering up, staying in the shade, and using sunscreen regularly and consistently. However, essential oils can also be used to combat free radicals and singlet oxygen caused by sun damage. Consider the following study, available on PubMed, which examines the effects of Myrrh essential oil on skin physiology in relation to UV irradiation.

Study 2 – Sun Protection

"Squalene is a component of sebum. Both are directly exposed to the external environment and play a key role in skin physiology. They are particularly prone to photo oxidation during sun exposure. We studied the impact of two types of antioxidant on sebum squalene peroxidation by UV irradiation. The first type is free radical scavenger (Butyl hydroxyl toluene and olive extract rich in hydroxytyrosol). The second type is the essential oil of Commiphora Myrrha, a singlet oxygen quencher...Our results clearly show that essential oil of Commiphora

Myrrha provides the best protection against squalene peroxidation. These results demonstrate that squalene peroxidation during solar exposure is mainly because of singlet oxygen and not due to free radical attack. This suggests that sun care cosmetics should make use not only of free radical scavengers but also of singlet oxygen quenchers."

The study examined the antioxidant effects of Myrrh essential oil in relation to sun exposure, UV irradiation, and skin physiology. Myrrh essential oil provided significant protection against singlet oxygen, which causes damaging effects on a number of organic materials through sunlight. In this way, Myrrh is an anti-agent working against the peroxidation of squalene, which is a natural moisturizer and one of the most common lipids created by human skin cells. Peroxidation is when free radicals take electrons from cell membranes, which results in the oxidative degradation of lipids and significant cell damage. This causes a chain reaction, because whenever a normal cell is in contact with a radical, another radical is produced, which means the radicals begin to multiply at an exponential rate, the end result being carcinogenic or mutagenic. The results of the study indicate that Myrrh demonstrates potential in the arena of skin care and cosmetics when it comes to sun protection.

Reference & Photo Credit:
http://www.ncbi.nlm.nih.gov/pubmed/18489308]

Apart from the primary factors that contribute to aging skin – pollution, photo aging, genetics, and natural processes of aging – secondary factors include gravity, stress, facial movement (frowning, smiling, squinting, etc.), and obesity.

So what can you do to create a natural anti-aging regimen for your skin?

The following protocols will help prevent damage to the skin's layers, which will abate the skin's normal aging process.

- **Sleep** – get your beauty sleep; that is, 7.5-8 hours a night on average. Sleep provides a renewal period for the body and, in particular, the skin, by hydrating and balancing – hence, the dryness and bags under the eyes when you don't get enough sleep. A lack of sleep also results in cells that are more likely to become damaged and inflamed. Without the deep sleep recovery period, hyaluronic acid and collagen are broken down, stealing the glow and luster from your complexion, and also prompting or worsening other skin conditions, like acne, dermatitis, and immune-related skin issues, like psoriasis and eczema. Additionally, sleep enables the body better control over weight management, and a healthy diet and weight is good on the skin (for solid sleep, see insomnia protocols).
- **Eat** – a healthy and nutritious diet of lean proteins,

fruits and vegetables, and healthy fats will promote bright, beautiful skin. Some of the best foods for healthy skin are the following: oats, barley, and brown rice, which offer a natural plant chemical that soothes irritated skin, and they are also low-glycemic, which means they won't spike blood pressure and cause wrinkles and acne; oranges, Grapefruit, parsley, and tomatoes, which are water heavy, offering your skin hydration and, in many cases, providing the body with vitamins and minerals that promote collagen, maintaining supple skin; avocados, walnuts, macadamia nut oil, and olive oil, which offer healthy fat that enables skin hydration and the absorption of much needed nutrients and vitamins; Brussel sprouts, kale, broccoli, cauliflower, and collard greens are chock full of vitamins A and C, which help prevent sun damage and strengthen collagen, respectively; lean beef, chicken, tofu, beans, and eggs provides protein, which is needed for skin health; and salmon, sardines, walnuts, mackerel, milk, and flaxseed all provide the omega-3 fats, which prevent skin cancer cells from increasing and spreading.

- **Sun** – as sun damage is one of the primary causes of premature skin aging, protecting yourself from the sun via a number of methods is a measure you should take to prevent skin damage. This includes seeking shade, particularly between the hours of 10 a.m. and 2 p.m.; covering up whenever possible with skirts, pants, long sleeves, hats, sunglasses, etc.;

skipping the tanning beds or sunlamps, which expose you to the same harmful UV rays as direct sunlight; and of course, using a water-resistant sunscreen regularly and generously, of SPF 30 or higher (see <u>sunscreen</u> recipe).

- **Maintenance** – wash the dirt and grime that accumulates on the face twice daily with a mild cleanser and warm water. Be gentle and avoid scrubbing, which can damage and inflame. Apply a moisturizer mixed with essential oils regularly to the skin (see <u>moisturizer</u> recipe). This will provide your dry skin with the hydration and antioxidants it needs to thrive, protect against signs of aging, and maintain its youthful appearance.

- **Avoid Bad Habits** – smoking, as mentioned, introduces toxins into the body which lead to a dull and dry complexion, leathery skin, premature wrinkles, and a loss of elasticity and firmness in the skin. Stop smoking and avoid excessive alcohol consumption in order to prevent these toxins from entering the body (see <u>addiction</u> protocols).

Essential Oil Protocols

Acne

Description:

Acne forms as a result of excess sebum, or dirt, clogging up the skin's pores. When the pores are clogged, bacteria can form and accumulate, become infected and inflamed, and produce pimples and acne. Acne is exacerbated during the teenage years due in part to hormonal fluctuation, and can also be influenced by cosmetics, excess moisture, diet, stress, and certain medications.

Application:

Cleanse your skin as normal, then combine 3-4 drops of your choice essential oil with 3-5 drops of carrier oil, and apply lightly to the affected area. Let oils absorb into the skin.

Recommended Oils:

Topical Blend, Thyme, Sandalwood, Tea Tree, Lemongrass, Lemon, Juniper Berry, Geranium, Cleansing Blend, Cedarwood

Other Natural Protocols:

Apple cider vinegar can also serve as a natural antifungal and antibacterial to eliminate acne blemishes. Use a Q-tip to apply topically seVeral times daily.

Addiction

Description:

Addiction to substances including tobacco, drugs, alcohol, pharmaceuticals, foods high in sugar, or to behaviors including sex, gambling, or gaming, results in adverse physical, mental, and emotional issues caused by the dependency to the substance or behavior. Physical symptoms of withdrawal may include nausea, cravings, irritability, or headaches, while emotional/psychological issues may include anxiety, guilt, and hopelessness.

Application:

• **Tobacco or sugar cravings** – for tobacco cravings, place a couple drops of Cinnamon in your drinking water. For sugar cravings, do the same with the Metabolic Blend or Grapefruit. Take orally whenever you feel a craving coming on.

• **Others** – for other dependencies, use an inhaler filled with the essential oil of your choice according to the dependency listed below. Inhale whenever necessary.

Recommended Oils:

Alcohol: Rosemary, Helichrysum, Cleansing Blend, Calming Blend

Anxiety: Ylang Ylang, Lavender, Grounding Blend, Calming Blend

Caffeine: Metabolic Blend, Basil

Cravings: Peppermint, Grounding Blend, Grapefruit, Clove, Cinnamon, Cilantro, Calming Blend

Drugs: Roman Chamomile, Grapefruit, Cleansing Blend, Calming Blend

Food: Metabolic Blend, Grapefruit

Marijuana: Basil

Sugar: Metabolic Blend, Grapefruit, Cleansing Blend, Calming Blend

Tobacco: Protective Blend, Black Pepper, Clove

Withdrawal: Wild Orange, Sandalwood, Marjoram, Lavender, Grapefruit

Other Natural Protocols:

Consider other essential oil-based products, like Basic Vitality Supplements (LLV). For alcoholics, try supplementing your protocol with vitamin B1 (thiamine), as most alcoholics are deficient in this vitamin.

Air Quality

Description:

The air you breathe can carry harmful agents, such as environmental pollutants and airborne pathogens. Limiting the oxidants that enter the body will benefit overall health. Aspects that increase levels of outdoor and indoor pollutants are extreme weather and improper ventilation.

Application:

• Airborne pathogens – diffuse essential oils throughout the home (Lemon, Respiratory Blend, Cleansing Blend, and Protective Blend are recommended).

• Ventilation – add a few drops of Protective Blend to filters in your homes Heater/AC duct system.

Recommended Oils:

Sandalwood, Respiratory Blend, Protective Blend, Peppermint, Tea Tree, Lemon, Lavender, Eucalyptus, and Cleansing Blend

Other Natural Protocols:

In case of outdoor pollutants, always keep the windows closed when levels are high. In case of indoor pollutants, eliminate the source, provide good ventilation, and use air filters or cleaners.

Antioxidants

Description:

Anything high in antioxidants – whether fruit, beans, or essential oils – is a powerful advocate for your body. Antioxidants both protect against free radicals and repair their damage. What are free radicals? Free radicals are destructive chemicals that invade your body, produced by substances both inside and out. Some free radicals (oxidants) form through normal bodily reactions, like inflammation, metabolism, and aerobic respiration. Other free radicals form outside the body, but enter it due to exposure. These include harmful pollutants, toxins, smoking, alcohol, X-rays, and UV rays, to name a few. Although our bodies produce their own antioxidants, these often become damaged as we grow older; thus, introducing antioxidants into our bodies allows these nutrients and enzymes to assist in chemical reactions which destroy the oxidants or free radicals.

Application:

Add 8 drops of your chosen essential oil to a capsule (Clove is suggested) and take internally once a week.

Recommended Oils:

White Fir, Thyme, Soothing Blend, Rosemary, Respiratory Blend, Protective Blend, Peppermint, Oregano, Tea Tree, Helichrysum, Frankincense, Clove, Cleansing Blend, Cinnamon

Other Natural Protocols:

Consider essential oil-based products, such as Basic Vitality Supplements (LLV). Other oils, like coconut, olive, and grapeseed oil, are also great sources of antioxidants.

Bags under Eyes

Description:

Bags under the eyes may be the result of seVeral causes, including allergies, water retention, overconsumption of alcohol, inactivity, or lack of sleep. In order to combat this issue, apply the appropriate protocol in accordance with the root cause.

Application:

Combine your chosen oil with virgin coconut oil in the designated dilution ratio. Apply topically below the eyes at night and in the morning. Be careful not to get oil in the eye.

Recommended Oils:

Sandalwood, Myrrh, Geranium, Frankincense, and Cypress

Other Natural Protocols:

Anti-Aging Moisturizer and Tightening Serum may both work to tone and tighten the skin. You might also try using a neti pot, which drains and flushes out excess moisture due to sinuses or allergies.

Chapped/Dry Skin

Description:

A number of issues can cause your skin to become dry or chapped, most having to do with a lack of moisture in the derma. Winter weather – which lacks in humidity – moisture-robbing body products, aging, or health conditions may be the root cause of the problem.

Application:

Dilute your chosen essential oil according to the dilution ratio with virgin coconut oil and apply topically (for Myrrh, 12-30 drops per ounce of coconut oil).

Recommended Oils:

Ylang Ylang, Metabolic Blend, Sandalwood, Patchouli, Peppermint, Oregano, Myrrh, Lemon, Lavender, Helichrysum, Grapefruit, Geranium, Frankincense, Cypress

Other Natural Protocols:

A Honey or yogurt rub will provide extra moisture to your skin. Apply either to the affected areas, leave on for 10 minutes, then shower as normal.

Inflammation

Description:

Inflammation is an immune system response with the intent to protect the body against invasive sources, including infections. There is acute inflammation – short-lived inflammation occurring immediately as a response to an irritant, strain, wound, or infection – and chronic inflammation – which is systemic and persistent. Inflammation may result in pain, heat, redness, swelling, and even immobility.

Application:

Dilute your chosen essential oil accordingly (Frankincense, Myrrh, and Helichrysum are suggested) with a carrier oil and apply topically to the affected area whenever needed.

Recommended Oils:

Peppermint, Myrrh, Lavender, Helichrysum, Ginger, Frankincense, Eucalyptus, and Basil

Other Natural Protocols:

For chronic inflammation, consider using the Basic Vitality Supplements (LLV) alongside a healthy and balanced diet. Ginger also helps reduce inflammation. Combine equal parts Ginger juice, Honey, and Pomegranate juice in a glass jug and consume one tablespoon 2-3 times daily.

Insomnia

Description:

Insomnia occurs when, due to unusual sleep patterns, a person cannot get the rest required to function properly. Insomnia can be caused by anxiety, stress, or caffeine/alcohol consumption, and includes an inability to fall asleep, stay asleep, or experience rest while sleeping. If insomnia occurs for seVeral weeks, the lack of sleep can have serious consequences, including chronic pain, restless leg syndrome, indigestion, and depression.

Application:

For internal application, place 1-3 drops of Clary Sage under the tongue before bedtime. For aromatic application, diffuse your chosen oil throughout the room (Calming Blend and Lavender are suggested) or place 2-3 drops in your hands and rub lightly across your pillow. For topical application, dilute your chosen oil accordingly (Lavender, Calming Blend, or equal parts Lavender/Lemon are suggested) and massage the feet. You might also try adding seVeral drops to a warm bath, disperse, and soak for twenty minutes.

Recommended Oils:

Ylang Ylang, Wild Orange, Rosemary, Roman Chamomile, Marjoram, Lavender, Frankincense, Clary Sage, and Calming Blend

Other Natural Protocols:

Mash up a banana and combine with 1 teaspoon cumin powder. Eat the mixture before going to sleep.

Oily Skin

Description:

Oily skin is the result of excess sebum and is often caused by stress, humid weather, diet, cosmetic use, or hormone fluctuation.

Application:

Add a couple drops of your chosen oil (Tea Tree or Peppermint are recommended) to a cotton swab and dab onto face. Allow the oil to absorb into the skin. Wash as normal.

Recommended Oils:

Ylang Ylang, Metabolic Blend, Sandalwood, Patchouli, Peppermint, Oregano, Myrrh, Lemon, Lavender, Helichrysum, Grapefruit, Geranium, Frankincense, Cypress

Other Natural Protocols:

Apply Aloe Vera gel topically, dabbing on the face or other affected area 2-3 times daily. Let air dry. Aloe Vera will absorb the oil and clear clogged pores. Store in the refrigerator to keep it cool.

Stress

Description:

Stress occurs naturally when the body reacts physically, mentally, and emotionally to difficult, tense, or unknown situations. Stress occurs in three stages: alarm, resistance, and exhaustion. Initially, the body responds to stress by producing adrenalin, which triggers the fight-or-flight response. Next, the body attempts to adapt if the stressor recurs. If the body is not able to cope with the stressor, it will become depleted by the demands placed upon it, which can result in mental or physical disorders, including depression, sleep issues, emotional instability, and even digestive and cardiovascular conditions.

Application:

Dilute your chosen oil (Patchouli, Wild Orange, Grounding Blend, Calming Blend, and Tension Blend are recommended) with a carrier oil according to its dilution ratio and apply topically in a full-body massage, hand or foot massage. You may also diffuse throughout the home, use the cup and inhale technique, or add a few drops to your bath and disperse.

Recommended Oils:

Ylang Ylang, Wild Orange, Thyme, Tension Blend, Rosemary, Patchouli, Marjoram, Lemon, Lavender, Joyful Blend, Invigorating Blend, Grounding Blend, Grapefruit, Geranium, Frankincense, Clary Sage, Calming Blend, Basil

Other Natural Protocols:

You might also consider essential-oil based products like Basic Vitality Supplements (LLV) or Massage Blend technique. To support mental and emotional balance, always maintain a healthy diet and eating habits. Fish oil is rich in omega-3 fatty acids and can help stimulate hormone production, nerve tissue health, and brain functionality. For the proper dosage on fish oil supplements, consult your doctor.

Sun Care

Description:

Sunburns occur due to ultraviolet radiation scorching the top layer of the skin. Most often, sunburns are first-degree burns, but they can also be mild second-degree burns if blistering results. Symptoms include pain, redness, and the skin feels hot to the touch.

Application:

Sunscreen – a moderate sunscreen can be made by filling a 2-ounce spray bottle with 60 drops each of Lavender and Helichrysum and topping it off with fractionated coconut oil. Use as normal.

General sunburn care – combine 20 drops each of Frankincense and Lavender with 1-ounce fractionated coconut oil in a small glass jar or bottle. Apply topically to the affected area 2-4 times daily.

Recommended Oils:

Sandalwood, Roman Chamomile, Peppermint, Tea Tree, Lavender, Helichrysum, and Frankincense

Other Natural Protocols:

Use sunscreen regularly. Aloe Vera has anti-inflammatory properties. Apply it topically to the sunburn and allow it to air dry.

Sun Spots

Description:

Sunspots can be caused by a fungus called tinea versicolor.

Application:

Dilute your chosen essential oil according to its appropriate ratio (Topical Blend is suggested) and apply to the affected area once daily, until the sun spots have vanished.

Recommended Oils:

Ylang Ylang, Metabolic Blend, Sandalwood, Patchouli, Peppermint, Oregano, Myrrh, Lemon, Lavender, Helichrysum, Grapefruit, Geranium, Frankincense, Cypress

Other Natural Protocols:

Though it may irritate sensitive skin, hydroquinone will help fade sun spots. Less irritating options include vitamin C, licorice extract, kojic acid, and alpha-arbutin. Try different combinations and layering of each substance.

Common Skin-aging Issues & Essential Oil Protocols

As one of the most visible signs of aging, skin changes – such as sagging skin and wrinkles – increase as the years pass by, no matter which preventative measures you have taken. No elixir of life will keep us youthful, but the speed at which our skin ages is indicative of how well we have taken care of our skin and, of course, of the wear-and-tear placed upon it through environmental factors and our own lifestyle choices.

Natural skin changes that accompany aging include rougher, more fragile, and more transparent skin, due to the flattening of the connective layer between the epidermis and dermis, and the thinning of the epidermis itself. The skin also becomes more susceptible to lesion development and bruising, resulting from thinner blood vessel walls and benign tumors. Additionally, skin tags, warts, and other growths become more prevalent in aging skin.

The slackening of the skin is due to the loss of elasticity. Moreover, aging below the skin's layers contributes to changes above the surface. For instance, the loss of bone around the chin and mouth produces a puckering in the skin, and the loss of fat in the chin, nose, cheeks, temples, and around the eyes produces skin looseness and a bony appearance.

Most other age-related skin issues are due to the thinning of the epidermis and the reduction in the number of melanocytes (pigment cells) in the skin. Due to this reduction the melanocytes which remain grow larger, causing the skin to become translucent, paler, and thinner in appearance, while liver spots, or age spots, are more apt to show up in areas of the skin that have been exposed to the sun.

The leathery appearance in some aging skin – which largely occurs in those who have spent a lot of time in the outdoors – is caused by weather-beating and sun exposure. These factors impact the strength and elasticity in the skin's connective tissue, producing elastosis.

Skin dryness and itchiness increases as we age, because the sebaceous glands produce less oil and provide less moisture to the skin. This often happens in women after menopause and in men after the age of 80.

Skin injury increases, and the body's ability to regulate body temperature decreases, due to the thinning of the skin layers and the subcutaneous fat layer, which generally provides insulation, padding, and added protection. The natural insulation protects against hypothermia, so the thinning of it makes older folks more susceptible to cold. Moreover, the fat layer also helps absorb certain medications, so the loss of it may impact the effectiveness of these medications. Regulation of the body's temperature is also influenced by sweat. As the body ages, less sweat is produced by the sweat glands, and so it is harder for the body to cool itself, resulting in a higher risk of heat stroke or overheating.

The skin is also more susceptible to pressure ulcers because of this loss of subcutaneous fat, coupled with inactivity, and deficiencies in nutrition.

All of this combined, means that aging skin is less capable of repairing itself than young, healthy skin. In fact, wounds may take four times longer to heal, which then amounts to a higher risk of infection and pressure ulcers. Other health issues that are associated with aging – such as a less effective immune system and changes in blood vessels – also impact the rate and quality of healing.

Essential oils can support many of these issues. Certain oils can reduce the appearance of wrinkles and sunspots by strengthening the skin's layers and promoting elasticity. Other oils can speed the healing process of scrapes and bruises, while still others will support the natural degeneration of nerves.

Essential Oil Protocols

Abscess

Description:

Abscesses are often caused by bacteria, parasites, infection, or foreign substances that create a buildup of white blood cells within the body. These excess cells and other substances produce pus, surrounded by irritation and redness. Abscesses can form in the skin, teeth, the liver, brain or rectum, and are more common in folks with weakened immune systems.

Application:

• Tooth abscess – add 2-4 drops of the essential oil of your choice (Oregano or Protective Blend are recommended) in a capsule and take daily until the pain ceases. Continue for 3 days after.

• Throat abscess – gargle 3 drops of your chosen oil (Lemon, Oregano, or Protective Blend are recommended) for 15-20 seconds and swallow.

• Skin Abscess – combine your chosen oil (Oregano, Protective Blend, and Tea Tree are recommended) with a carrier oil according to its specified dilution ratio and apply topically to the affected area every ½ hour.

Recommended Oils:

Roman Chamomile, Oregano, Protective Blend, Tea Tree, Lavender, Helichrysum, Frankincense, Clove, Cleansing Blend

Other Natural Protocols:

Apple cider vinegar can disinfect and relieve swelling for tooth abscesses. Swish in your mouth for several minutes and spit out.

Age Spots

Description:

Age spots, or liver spots, are common in those over 50 years of age and tend to develop on hands, arms, shoulders, the face, and other areas open to the sun. Age spots are flat and either black, brown, or tan. Though age spots are harmless and not cancerous, they can be unsightly on otherwise youthful-looking skin. For cosmetic reasons, many wish to eliminate age spots.

Application:

To get rid of age spots, dilute your chosen essential oil (recommended: Myrrh, Lavender, or Frankincense) in extra virgin coconut oil according to the appropriate ratio and apply topically to the affected area each day.

Recommended Oils:

Ylang Ylang, Metabolic Blend, Sandalwood, Patchouli, Peppermint, Oregano, Myrrh, Lemon, Lavender, Helichrysum, Grapefruit, Geranium, Frankincense, Cypress

Other Natural Protocols:

Though it may irritate sensitive skin, hydroquinone will help fade brown spots. Less irritating options include vitamin C, licorice extract, kojic acid, and alpha-arbutin. Try different combinations and layering of each substance. You might also try other natural essential oils-based products, such as Basic Vitality Supplements (LLV), Topical Blend,

Detoxification Blend, GI cleansing Formula, Anti-Aging Blend, or Probiotic Defense Formula.

Bed Sores

Description:

Bed sores are pressure ulcers; in other words, injuries that result from consistent pressure being applied to a limited area, which often occurs when someone is confined to the bed for a prolonged period. The pressure most commonly occurs in the hip, buttocks, tailbone, heel, and/or ankle, where the bone influences the pressure on contact. Older individuals are more sensitive to bedsores as their skin is thinner and, if left untreated, the sores can open and become infected.

Application:

Dilute your chosen oil (blends of equal parts Lavender and Helichrysum or Rosemary and Tea Tree are suggested) accordingly with a carrier oil and apply topically to the affected area up to three times daily.

Recommended Oils:

Ylang Ylang, Rosemary, Myrrh, Tea Tree, Marjoram, Lavender, Frankincense, Helichrysum, Geranium, and Cypress

Other Natural Protocols:

Consider essential-oil based products, like Basic Vitality Supplements (LLV). Prevention with good nutrition, to assure healthy skin, is suggested. If your patient is confined to a reclining position, always reposition them three or more times each day so that prolonged pressure is avoided. Also consider administering saline solution to clean the sores (a pinch of baking soda and one teaspoon of non-iodized salt in a quart of distilled water). Apply twice a day and bandage.

Bruises/Hematomas

Description:

Bruises occur when blood vessels break near the skin's surface, when the body is either hit hard or strained in some way, resulting in a discolored area and possible swelling or pain. A hematoma is a collection of blood outside of a blood vessel and can occur in any of the body's organs. Though slight bruising is not a serious issue, severe bruising can indicate a more serious problem within the body.

Application:

• Immediate application – dilute your chosen oil accordingly (Helichrysum or a Cypress/Lavender blend are suggested) and apply topically to the affected area, applying a cold compress over the bruise every 15 minutes, leaving the compress on for 15 minutes.

• Later application – after 6-24 hours, increase blood circulation by applying 1-3 drops of Helichrysum neat to the affected area. Alternate hot and cold compresses.

Recommended Oils:

Soothing Blend, Rosemary, Myrrh, Lemongrass, Lavender, Helichrysum, Geranium, Fennel, and Cypress

Other Natural Protocols:

Apply a cold herbal tea compress. To prepare, add a teaspoon each of dried Lavender flowers and dried

Chamomile flowers in a cup of hot water, let steep for 15 minutes, strain and refrigerate. Dip your compress into the tea and apply to the affected area, leaving on for 10 minutes. Repeat a few times daily.

Heat Exhaustion/Heat Stroke

Description:

Heat exhaustion occurs when the body's ability to cool itself is inadequate to the amount of physical exertion, due to extremely hot or humid climates, dehydration, or sweating. Symptoms include an increase in temperature, flushed face, weakness, and disorientation. Heat stroke occurs if the temperature rises above 104 F. Seek medical attention, as symptoms of heat stroke also include increased heart rate, vomiting, diarrhea, convulsions/seizures, unconsciousness, and flushed color in other body parts.

Application:

Add a couple drops of Peppermint to a cool, damp cloth and apply to the forehead. For topical application, apply 2-3 drops of Peppermint to the chest, the neck, the back of the neck, and the soles of the feet. Use the cup and inhale method and, if the body temperature rises extremely, give the patient a sponge bath.

Recommended Oils:

Peppermint and Lavender

Other Natural Protocols:

First and foremost, always move the person to a shady and cool area, rehydrate them with cool beverages (avoid carbonated drinks and alcohol), and place them in a restful position.

Itchy Skin

Description:

Itchy skin can be caused by a number of factors, including dryness, nervous disorders, rashes, internal diseases, allergic reactions, drugs, or pregnancy.

Application:

Dilute your chosen oil (Lavender, Patchouli, or Peppermint are particularly recommended) with a carrier oil and apply topically to the affected area.

Recommended Oils:

Ylang Ylang, Metabolic Blend, Sandalwood, Patchouli, Peppermint, Oregano, Myrrh, Lemon, Lavender, Helichrysum, Grapefruit, Geranium, Frankincense, Cypress

Other Natural Protocols:

If itchiness is caused by toxins, cleanse using Probiotic Defense Formula or GI Cleansing Formula. Also consider converting temporarily to a vegan diet with green smoothies. Extra-virgin olive oil also fortifies the skin, as it is rich in antioxidants and vitamin E. Combine with Honey in equal parts and apply topically to the affected area several times a day.

Sagging Skin

Description:

Sagging or loose skin results from aging. As the skin no longer has as much elastin to bounce back, this disallows the underlying skin to tighten quickly enough.

Application:

Dilute your chosen oil accordingly (Helichrysum is suggested) with a carrier oil and apply topically to the affected area.

Recommended Oils:

Ylang Ylang, Metabolic Blend, Sandalwood, Patchouli, Peppermint, Oregano, Myrrh, Lemon, Lavender, Helichrysum, Grapefruit, Geranium, Frankincense, Cypress

Other Natural Protocols:

Consider essential oil-based products, like the Anti-Aging Moisturizer, Metabolic Blend, and the Metabolic Blend Kit. Also consider combining the Metabolic Blend with Grapefruit oil and applying topically. Additionally, consistently tone and condition your areas of concern. For sagging of the facial skin, whisk 1-2 egg whites into a foam and apply it to the affected areas of the neck and face, allowing it to sit for 20 minutes. Rinse off with cool water.

Scars

Description:

Scars occur after a wound from disease, surgery, or an accident repairs itself, causing a visible blemish in the skin that usually diminishes over time.

Application:

Add 6 drops each of Frankincense, Lavender, and Helichrysum to a roller bottle and add 6 capsules of vitamin E oil. Fill the remainder with extra virgin coconut oil and apply consistently up to 3 times a day.

Recommended Oils:

White Fir, Soothing Blend, Sandalwood, Rose, Myrrh, Lavender, Helichrysum, Geranium, Frankincense, and Eucalyptus

Other Natural Protocols:

Warm a tbsp. of coconut oil in the microwave for a few seconds and gently massage into the affected area in a circular motion several times daily.

Skin Tags

Description:

Skin tags are small flaps of tissue hanging from, and connected to, the skin. They are found in the armpit, the groin area, or on the neck, back, and chest. They can be the result of skin rubbing against skin, weight gain, aging, or viruses.

Application:

Dilute your chosen essential oil according to its appropriate ratio (Frankincense or Oregano are suggested) and apply to the tag up to three times daily, until the tag is removed.

Recommended Oils:

Ylang Ylang, Metabolic Blend, Sandalwood, Patchouli, Peppermint, Oregano, Myrrh, Lemon, Lavender, Helichrysum, Grapefruit, Geranium, Frankincense, Cypress

Other Natural Protocols:

Skin tags can be removed naturally by cutting with a scalpel or scissors or cryosurgery (freezing). Before you do so, consult a dermatologist. You can also try dabbing apple cider vinegar on the tag with a cotton swab, leaving on for three hours, and rinsing with warm water. Follow this protocol three times a day for 2-4 weeks.

Skin Ulcerations

Description:

Skin ulcerations include any type of skin condition that involves open sores.

Application:

For general skin ulcerations, apply Lavender neat to the affected area. For more serious ulcerations, combine Helichrysum and Frankincense and apply topically to the affected area twice daily.

Recommended Oils:

Topical Blend, Rosemary, Roman Chamomile, Myrrh, Lavender, Helichrysum, Geranium, Frankincense, Eucalyptus, Detoxification Blend, Cypress, Clove, and Bergamot

Other Natural Protocols:

Consider essential oil-based products, like Detoxification Blend, Detoxification Complex, GI Cleansing Formula/Probiotic Defense Formula, and Digestive Enzyme Complex. Also consider administering saline solution to clean the sores (a pinch of baking soda and one teaspoon of non-iodized salt in a quart of distilled water). Apply twice a day and bandage.

Varicose Veins

Description:

Varicose veins occur when the veins become weak through pressure or time and grow visibly enlarged and twisted. This often occurs in the lower extremities and can be influenced by age, continuous standing, being overweight, and pregnancy. Severity of the issue varies from mild spider veins to severe varicose veins, even further to deep vein thrombosis. Other symptoms include, pain, itching, swelling, discoloration, and skin changes.

Application:

Combine 30 drops Cypress, 20 drops Lavender, and 10 drops of any citrus oil, with 2 ounces coconut oil in a small glass jar or bottle. Apply topically to the affected area morning and night every day.

Recommended Oils:

Peppermint, Lemongrass, Lemon, Lavender, Invigorating Blend, Helichrysum, Geranium, Cypress, and Citrus Oils

Other Natural Protocols:

Massage apple cider vinegar gently into the area of concern, morning and night, every day for several months.

Warts

Description:

Warts are the result of a viral infection occurring in the skin's outer layer, with the consistency of a small circular scab growth. Warts typically occur on the feet or hands and are contagious upon contact. Warts have different names, depending upon location, such as common warts (typical raised circles ¼ inch in diameter), plantar warts (soles of the feet), filiform warts (around the chin, nose, and mouth), molluscum warts (pimple-like, and on the legs, arms, or trunk, flat warts (flatter than the common wart and occurring on the legs, arms, or face), periungual warts (bumps around toenails and fingernails), genital warts (sexual transmitted disease occurring in the area of the genitals).

Application:

Common, flat, plantar, and periungual warts – dilute your chosen oil accordingly (1 drop each of Oregano and Frankincense is suggested) with a carrier oil and apply topically to the affected area up to three times daily for 2-4 weeks. Continue protocol for a week after removal.

Molluscum warts – dilute your chosen oil accordingly (Protective Blend, Lavender, Cleansing Blend, Tea Tree, or Oregano are suggested) with a carrier oil and apply topically to the affected area up to three times daily for 2-4 weeks. Continue protocol for a week after removal.

Recommended Oils:

Thyme, Protective Blend, Oregano, Tea Tree, Lemon, Frankincense, Cypress, Clove, Cleansing Blend, and Cinnamon.

Other Natural Protocols:

Apply petroleum jelly around the wart. Crush the clove of garlic to make a paste and apply topically to the wart, covering it over with a bandage. Let sit for 20 minutes, remove the bandage, and repeat twice daily for a week, after which the wart should blister and fall off.

Wounds & Cuts

Description:

Wounds and cuts occur when the skin breaks. There may be bleeding and the severity of the wound or cut varies.

Application:

• Clean the wound – apart from soap and water, a wound can be cleaned with a spritz of Protective Blend or Tea Tree.

• Stopping bleeding – dilute your chosen oil accordingly (Helichrysum and Lemon are suggested) with a carrier oil and apply topically to the wound or cut to aid in blood clotting.

Recommended Oils:

Protective Blend, Myrrh, Tea Tree, Lemon, Lavender, Helichrysum, Geranium, Frankincense, and Cleansing Blend

Other Natural Protocols:

For minor cuts or wounds, the basic steps include applying pressure to stop the bleeding, cleaning the wound, applying antibiotic, bandaging the wound, and monitoring the wound for infection. Honey can also work as a natural antiseptic. After cleaning a wound or cut with soap and water, apply Honey over the affected area and cover with a bandage. Also consider essential oil-based products, like Protective Blend hand wipes.

Wrinkles

Description:

Wrinkles are often caused by smiling and frowning and other physicalities that manipulate the skin. They accumulate as we age.

Application:

A combined protocol calls for tightening serum (information on serum made with Sandalwood, Frankincense, and Myrrh) and moisturizing skin lotion (information on lotion made with Geranium, jasmine, Frankincense, and Lavender)

Recommended Oils:

Ylang Ylang, Metabolic Blend, Sandalwood, Patchouli, Peppermint, Oregano, Myrrh, Lemon, Lavender, Helichrysum, Grapefruit, Geranium, Frankincense, Cypress

Other Natural Protocols:

Along with moisturizer, massage olive oil regularly onto the skin, in order to repair and regenerate skin cells.

Chapter 2:
Bone, Muscle & Joint Health

The skeletal structure, which supports the body, is composed of joints and bones, which allow for flexibility of movement. The joint is a cushion of cartilage with synovial membranes and fluid surrounding it. Supported by this cushion the bones do not rub up against each other and wear away. Muscles provide the skeleton with strength and inertia to move, while the brain coordinates their efforts.

As with skin and hair changes, aging bones, joints, and muscles produce changes in walking gait and posture. This is because the muscles and joints are weakened as we age, leading to slower movements. However, there are some anti-aging precautions everyone can take when it comes to muscle, bone, and joint health. In order to combat the body's daily wear-and-tear and decelerate aging, consider the following natural protocols, and support these protocols with regular essential oil use, according to your body's needs.

Anti-aging Bone, Muscle & Joint Care 101: Essential Oils & Preventative Protocols

Our bones are the storage structures for such minerals as phosphorous and calcium; these minerals provide bones the strength to support movement and protect our heart, brain, and other organs from external injury. It is important to support bone strength as natural aging processes reduce the minerals in bones, weakening them and causing greater risk of fracture.

One of the best ways to prevent issues with bones, muscles, and joints is, of course, diet and exercise. A balanced diet that promotes the right vitamins, minerals, and nutrients will prevent bone, muscle, and joint decay. Calcium, and vitamin D in particular, are necessary for healthy bones. Daily consumption of 1,200 mg of calcium and 400-800 units of vitamin D are recommended for postmenopausal women and men over 65-years-old. Regular moderate exercise can promote flexibility, strength, and balance of muscles and bones.

Strength training is key to preventing muscular degradation. Strength training involves using weights to progressively increase resistance so that key muscle groups must generate increased force. Working key muscle groups can improve muscle mass, body composition, and protect against a number of conditions that occur with aging, including sarcopenia. In addition to strength training, vitamin E has been shown to reduce muscle damage by combating oxidative stress created by free radicals following exercise.

Some carrier oils – like coconut, olive, and jojoba – are good sources of the antioxidant vitamin E as well, while essential oils themselves, can reduce oxidative stress. Consider the following study published by the *Asian Pacific Journal of Tropical Medicine*, in which the antioxidant effects of Marjoram essential oil were examined.

Study 3 – Antioxidant Properties

"To investigate the effects of prallethrin on renal dysfunction biomarkers, antioxidant enzyme activities and lipid peroxidation (LPO) in rats and the protective effect of Origanum majorana essential oil…We can conclude that prallethrin induced oxidative damage and renal toxicity in male rat. The administration of essential oil provided significant protection against prallethrin-induced oxidative stress, biochemical changes and histopathological damage."

The study's objective was to evaluate Marjoram essential oil's antioxidant effects. In the trial, four groups of rats were used; one receiving plain olive oil, another olive oil and prallethrin (a common insecticide), another prallethrin and Marjoram essential oil, and the last, the essential oil combined with olive oil. The applications were provided twice a day for 28 days, after which the effects on lipid peroxidation were evaluated. Lipid peroxidation is when free radicals take electrons from cell membranes, which results in the oxidative degradation of lipids and significant cell damage. This causes a chain reaction, because whenever a normal cell is in contact with a radical, another radical is produced, which means the radicals begin to multiply at an exponential rate, the end result being carcinogenic or mutagenic. Marjoram essential oil demonstrated natural antioxidant properties, inhibiting the free radicals from damaging cell walls and multiplying.

Reference:
http://www.ncbi.nlm.nih.gov/pubmed/25312175]

http://ac.els-cdn.com/S1995764514602820/1-s2.0-S1995764514602820-main.pdf?_tid=355bbd9e-d089-11e4-b460-00000aacb362&acdnat=1427025025_f612698f97f1ae2ba8d2779630e7c88b]

While resistance training is an excellent preventative measure to condition your muscles to age gracefully, always accompany your exercise regimen with adequate vitamins and minerals to support your output, including vitamin E. Those who are older should strength train in moderation, as the free radicals produced from resistance training have the potential to further muscle damage.

Below are a few essential oil protocols to support muscle maintenance and measures to combat oxidative stress.

Essential Oil Protocols

Antioxidants

Description:

Anything high in antioxidants – whether fruit, beans, or essential oils – is a powerful advocate for your body. Antioxidants both protect against free radicals and repair their damage. What are free radicals? Free radicals are destructive chemicals that invade your body, produced by substances both inside and out. Some free radicals (oxidants) form through normal bodily reactions, like inflammation, metabolism and aerobic respiration. Other free radicals form outside the body, but enter it due to exposure. These include harmful pollutants, toxins, smoking, alcohol, X-rays, and UV rays, to name a few. Although our bodies produce their own antioxidants, these often become damaged as we grow older; thus, introducing antioxidants into our bodies allows these nutrients and enzymes to assist in chemical reactions which destroy the oxidants or free radicals.

Application:

Add 8 drops of your chosen essential oil to a capsule (Clove is suggested) and take internally once a week.

Recommended Oils:

White Fir, Thyme, Soothing Blend, Rosemary,

Respiratory Blend, Protective Blend, Peppermint, Oregano, Tea Tree, Helichrysum, Frankincense, Clove, Cleansing Blend, Cinnamon

Other Natural Protocols:

Consider essential oil-based products, such as Basic Vitality Supplements (LLV). Other oils, like coconut, olive, and grapeseed oil, are also great sources of antioxidants.

Bone Health

Description:

Support strong bones and mineral retention through the following applications.

Application:

Dilute your chosen oil accordingly (Wintergreen, White Fir, or Soothing Blend are suggested) with a carrier oil and apply topically to the affected area and to the reflex points of the feet. For a routine application to strengthen bone health or for broken bones, dilute equal parts Cypress and Wintergreen (Eucalyptus or Smoothing Blend also work) accordingly and apply to the affected area before bed and in the morning do the same with a blend of Oregano, Grounding Blend, and Helichrysum or Frankincense.

Recommended Oils:

Wintergreen, White Fir, Thyme, Soothing Blend, Rosemary, Peppermint, Oregano, Lemon, Helichrysum, Grounding Blend, Geranium, Frankincense, Eucalyptus, Cypress, and Clove

Other Natural Protocols:

Consider essential oil-based products, like Bone Nutrient Lifetime Complex and Basic Vitality Supplements (LLV), which will provide the vitamins and minerals necessary for bone health. Exercise regularly and augment your nutritional protocol with calcium capsules. Prunes also help prevent fractures. Eat 2-3 prunes every day and, if you have reached an age where bones are weakening, increase your intake to 6-10 a day.

Muscle Pain & Maintenance

Description:

Muscle aches and pains are also known as myalgia and are often due to overexertion, certain medications, or are a symptom of a larger health concern, such as infection, disease, or stress disorders.

Application:

General – dilute your chosen oil accordingly (Peppermint is suggested) with a carrier oil and apply topically to the affected area. You may also consider a full-body massage for aches across several muscle regions, or a hot bath with your chosen oils.

Recommended Oils:

Wintergreen, Soothing Blend, Rosemary, Peppermint, Myrrh, Marjoram, Lemon, Lavender, Invigorating Blend, Ginger, Frankincense, Eucalyptus, and Birch

Other Natural Protocols:

Epsom salt offers magnesium, which helps ease muscle cramps and pain. Prepare a hot bath with 2 cups Epsom salt, disperse and soak for 20 minutes.

Common Bone- Muscle- and Joint- Aging Issues & Essential Oil Protocols

As people age bone density and mass decrease, particularly when calcium and other minerals are lost after menopause. The spine takes a hit as the discs which cushion the vertebrae grow thinner and lose fluid, making the trunk (the body's middle) grow shorter. The vertebrae also thin as the bones lose minerals, making the spine curve and compress, which sometimes results in bone spurs. This causes the stooped posture often seen in old age. The arm and leg bones become more brittle as well, leading to greater risk of breaks; and the foot arches are not as pronounced, resulting in a small reduction in height. All of this contributes to slower movement, less energy, and a shorter gait.

When it comes to the joints, many experience less flexibility and increased stiffness. This is due to a reduction in joint fluid and the erosion of cartilage as the joints create friction over time. This happens often in the hip and knee joints, as well as in the finger joints. Additionally, calcification occurs around some joints, creating hardened mineral deposits. This happens most often in the shoulder. Across many joints you can find inflammation, stiffness, and pain, increases as the joint structures break down. This may also lead to arthritis or deformity.

Muscle tissue loss, or atrophy, occurs naturally as we age, and the rate and severity of the loss is often hereditary. Changes in the muscle tissue include a deposit of fat and lipofuscin, which is a pigment related to aging. The fibers of the muscle shrink and the tissue is renewed at a slower rate. Tough fibrous tissue sometimes replaces the muscle tissue that is lost, as often occurs in the hands, making them bony and thin. These alterations in the muscle tissue, together with the alterations in the nervous system, influence the muscles' capacity to contract, contributing to their rigidity and loss of tone. With less muscle mass, endurance and strength are weakened, causing fatigue and exhaustion more regularly.

These common bone-, muscle-, and joint-aging issues lead to conditions like osteoporosis, which is particularly common in older women, as the bones are more brittle and, therefore, more likely to snap. Mobility often decreases with this condition as pain and compression fractures of the vertebrae inhibit movement. Loss of balance, instability, and muscle weakness also increase the risk of falling and possible breakage.

Additionally, joint conditions like osteoarthritis, can result in anything from mild stiffness to severe and debilitating pain. These changes in the muscles and joints also result in more frequent involuntary movements like muscle tremors.

Essential oils can help tone and strengthen muscles and provide general muscle maintenance. You can certainly use any of the previous protocols to support ongoing conditions. Additionally, some oils can reduce the pain and inflammation of arthritis, while others can support the healing of fractures, and still more can impede muscle tremors.

Essential Oil Protocols

Arthritis

Description:

Arthritis – including rheumatoid arthritis and osteoarthritis – involves inflammation of the joints, which can cause pain and some immobility or deformity of joints. Osteoarthritis inflammation is due to the cartilage of the contact surfaces of the bone degenerating. Rheumatoid arthritis is due to an autoimmune disease, whereby the connective tissue is attacked by the body, leading to deterioration of the cartilage.

Application:

For short-term pain relief dilute your chosen essential oil accordingly (Wintergreen, Birch, Peppermint and Soothing Blend are suggested) and apply topically to the affected area. You may also fill a bowl with hot water and add a few drops of essential oil; stir and soak your hands or feet for several minutes.

Recommended Oils:

Wintergreen, Vetiver, Soothing Blend, Sandalwood, Peppermint, Oregano, Myrrh, Marjoram, Lime, Lemon, Lavender, Ginger, German Chamomile, Geranium, Frankincense, Eucalyptus, and Birch

Other Natural Protocols:

Also consider essential oil-based products, like the GI Cleansing Formula and Basic Vitality Supplements (LLV). Apple cider vinegar can help relieve joint pain by expelling toxins that build up in the tissue. Add one teaspoon of apple cider vinegar and one of Honey to a cup of warm water and drink a glass every morning.

Back Pain

Description:

Back pain is generally related to conditions with the spinal column, including injury or disease of discs, vertebrae, or the spinal cord.

Application:

• Immediate relief – dilute your chosen oil accordingly (Birch, Wintergreen, and Soothing Blend are suggested) with a carrier oil and apply topically to the affected area. Apply a hot compress following application.

• Relax muscles – dilute your chosen oil accordingly (Marjoram, Roman Chamomile, Lime, and Massage Blend are suggested) with a carrier oil and apply topically to the affected area. Apply a hot compress following application.

• Regenerate tissue – dilute your chosen oil accordingly (Helichrysum, Frankincense, and Sandalwood are suggested) with a carrier oil and apply topically to the affected area up to three times daily. Apply a hot compress following application.

Recommended Oils:

Wintergreen, White Fir, Thyme, Soothing Blend, Sandalwood, Rosemary, Peppermint, Oregano, Myrrh, Marjoram, Lemon, Lavender, Grounding Blend, Eucalyptus, Cypress, Birch, and Basil

Other Natural Protocols:

Apple cider vinegar can help relieve pain by expelling toxins that build up in joint and muscle tissue. Add one teaspoon of apple cider vinegar and one of Honey to a cup of warm water and drink a glass every morning.

Broken Bones

Description:

Bone breaks or fractures occur when ligaments, tendons, or bones are crushed in injury. Such injuries may require surgery, plates, screws, and physical therapy. Symptoms include swelling, severe pain (especially in movement), nerve damage, and deformity. Fracture types include open fractures (where bone is exposed), stress fractures (overuse), comminuted fracture (fragmented fracture), spiral fracture (twisted bone), transverse fracture (right angle break), and greenstick fracture (diameter break).

Application:

• Pain – dilute your chosen oil accordingly (Soothing Blend and Wintergreen are suggested) and apply topically to affected area.

• Promote healing – dilute your chosen oil accordingly (recommendations: Birch (bone repair), Helichrysum and Marjoram (nerve and tissue regeneration/repair), Cypress (circulation), Lemongrass (ligament healing), White Fir (anti-inflammatory)) and apply topically to affected area up to three times daily.

Recommended Oils:

White Fir, Vetiver, Marjoram, Oregano, Lemongrass, Helichrysum, Ginger, Eucalyptus, Cypress, Clove, and Birch

Other Natural Protocols:

Consider using essential oil-based products, like the Basic Vitality Supplements (LLV). Prunes help prevent fractures. Eat 2-3 prunes every day and if you have reached an age where bones are weakening, then increase your intake to 6-10 a day.

Carpal Tunnel Syndrome

Description:

The carpal tunnel involves the flexor tendons in the wrist and fingers, and the tunnel that forms by the wrist bones and the transverse carpal ligament. Sensations are transferred to the three fingers and movement of the thumb through the median nerve. When carpal tunnel syndrome occurs as a result of arthritis, bone spurs, wrist injuries, repetition of movement, obesity, or pregnancy this median nerve is either numb or irritated, resulting in tingling, weakness, and pain.

Application:

• Pain – dilute your chosen oil accordingly (Soothing Blend and Wintergreen are suggested) with a carrier oil and apply topically to the affected area up to three times daily.

• Promoting healing – dilute your chosen oil accordingly (Massage Blend, Marjoram (muscle tissue), Frankincense, Helichrysum (nerve damage), Cypress (circulation), and Lemongrass (connective tissue) are suggested) with a carrier oil and apply topically to the affected area up to three times daily.

Recommended Oils:

Wintergreen, Soothing Blend, Oregano, Massage Blend, Marjoram, Lemongrass, Lavender, Helichrysum, Eucalyptus, Cypress, Clove, Birch, and Basil

Other Natural Protocols:

Apply a warm compress to the affected area for 5-7 minutes to relieve numbness and discomfort.

Exhaustion/Fatigue/Low Energy

Description:

Fatigue occurs either physically or mentally and can be caused by overexertion, low blood sugar, malnutrition, obesity, hypertension, hormonal imbalance, or psychological conditions, like depression and stress. Fatigue also may be indicative of a larger issue.

Application:

Diffuse your chosen oil throughout the home, or use the cup and inhale method, throughout the day. You can also start your day out right by adding a couple drops of stimulating oil to your feet after a morning shower (Peppermint is suggested). For other topical applications, dilute your chosen oil accordingly (Joyful Blend, Peppermint, or Rosemary are suggested) with a carrier oil and massage into the back of the neck, below the hairline.

Recommended Oils:

Wild Orange, White Fir, Rosemary, Peppermint, Lemon, Lavender, Joyful Blend, Invigorating Blend, Grapefruit, Frankincense, Eucalyptus, Cinnamon, Cassia, Calming Blend, Bergamot, and Basil

Other Natural Protocols:

Consider essential oil-based products, like Basic Vitality Supplements (LLV), GI Cleansing Formula, Probiotic Defense Formula, and Detoxification Blend. Eat a banana, which is full of vitamins and nutrients that promote energy, while combatting fatigue and dehydration. Also consider green tea, which helps boost energy and mental focus.

Joint Pain

Description:

Joint pain occurs when the joint is inflamed, resulting in either mild irritation or chronic debilitating pain. This can be caused by injury, disease, or overuse.

Application:

General care – dilute your chosen oil accordingly (Lavender, Soothing Blend, Peppermint, Wintergreen, Marjoram, or Frankincense are suggested) with a carrier oil and apply topically to affected area as needed. Also consider filling a basin or bathtub with warm water, adding and dispersing your chosen oil, and soaking the area of concern. If using compresses, alternate between hot and cold.

Pain – dilute your chosen oil accordingly (Rosemary, Ginger, Frankincense, Cypress, and Birch are suggested) with a carrier oil and apply topically to affected area as needed.

Warming – dilute your chosen oil accordingly (Cinnamon, Oregano, Clove, and Eucalyptus are suggested) with a carrier oil and apply topically to affected area as needed.

Recommended Oils:

Wintergreen, Soothing Blend, Rosemary, Peppermint, Oregano, Marjoram, Lavender, Ginger, Frankincense, Eucalyptus, Cypress, Clove, and Birch

Other Natural Protocols:

Consider essential oil-based products, like Soothing Blend Rub and Basic Vitality Supplements (LLV). Ginger also helps reduce inflammation. Combine equal parts Ginger juice, Honey, and Pomegranate juice in a glass jug and consume one tablespoon 2-3 times daily.

Knee Injuries/Pain

Description:

Knee pain can be caused by physical activity or injury, tears or strains, continual wear and tear, cysts (such as Baker's cyst), infections, diseases or disorders, including gout, rheumatoid arthritis, tendonitis, iliotibial band syndrome, lupus, or Osgood-Schlatter condition. The pain is usually caused by inflammation.

Application:

Circulation/warming – dilute your chosen oil accordingly (Clove, Cinnamon, Oregano, Eucalyptus, Grapefruit, and Peppermint are suggested) with a carrier oil and apply topically to the affected area.

General – dilute your chosen oil accordingly (Soothing Blend, Massage Blend, Lavender, Frankincense, Marjoram, Wintergreen, Lemongrass, and Peppermint are suggested) with a carrier oil and apply topically the affected area 2-3 times daily. Follow up with a hot compress.

Pain – see Pain protocol (Soothing Blend, Tension Blend, Wintergreen, White Fir, and Birch are suggested).

Tissue repair – dilute your chosen oil accordingly (Lemongrass, Helichrysum, and Frankincense are suggested) with a carrier oil and apply topically to the affected area.

Recommended Oils:

Wintergreen, Soothing Blend, Rosemary, Peppermint, Massage Blend, Marjoram, Lemongrass, Lavender, Grounding Blend, Ginger, Frankincense, and Cypress

Other Natural Protocols:

Consider essential oil-based products, like Basic Vitality Supplements (LLV). Ginger also helps reduce inflammation. Combine equal parts Ginger juice, Honey, and Pomegranate juice in a glass jug and consume one tablespoon 2-3 times daily.

Muscle Cramps/Spasms

Description:

Involuntary muscle cramps and spasms occur as a result of muscle contractions due to over-exercise, injury, nerve irritation, dehydration, or lack of nutrients. Spasms/cramps include issues like a charley horse, night cramps, or menstrual cramps. Certain conditions may also increase a person's susceptibility to cramps, such as pregnancy or dialysis. Stress, arthritis, and diuretics may also contribute to susceptibility.

Application:

Dilute your chosen oil accordingly (Soothing Blend, Massage Blend, and Tension Blend are suggested) with a carrier oil and massage into the affected area as needed. Follow up with a hot compress.

Recommended Oils:

Tension Blend, Soothing Blend, Roman Chamomile, Massage Blend, Marjoram, Lime, Lavender, Helichrysum, Geranium, and Cypress

Other Natural Protocols:

Consider essential oil-based products, like Basic Vitality Supplements (LLV). Epsom salt offers magnesium, which helps ease muscle cramps and pain. Prepare a hot bath with 2 cups Epsom salt, disperse and soak for 20 minutes.

Osteoporosis

Description:

Osteoporosis occurs in the bones due to insufficient levels of phosphate and calcium in the body, resulting in bone weakness, making them more susceptible to fractures. Two types of osteoporosis exist, primary osteoporosis (largely due to hormonal imbalance), and secondary osteoporosis (the minerals are lost due to side effects of disease or of taking certain medications). The disease may cause dowager's hump (stooped posture) and frequent fractures.

Application:

Dilute your chosen oil accordingly (Wintergreen, White Fir, or Soothing Blend are suggested) with a carrier oil and apply topically to the affected area, and to the reflex points of the feet. For a routine application to strengthen bone health or for broken bones, dilute equal parts Cypress and Wintergreen (Eucalyptus or Smoothing Blend also work) accordingly and apply to the affected area before bed and in the morning do the same with a blend of Oregano, Grounding Blend, and Helichrysum or Frankincense.

Recommended Oils:

Wintergreen, White Fir, Thyme, Soothing Blend, Rosemary, Peppermint, Oregano, Lemon, Helichrysum, Grounding Blend, Geranium, Frankincense, Eucalyptus, Cypress, and Clove

Other Natural Protocols:

Consider essential oil-based products, like Bone Nutrient Lifetime Complex and Basic Vitality Supplements (LLV), which will provide the vitamins and minerals necessary for bone health. Exercise regularly and augment your nutritional protocol with calcium capsules. Prunes also help prevent fractures. Eat 2-3 prunes every day and, if you have reached an age where bones are weakening, increase your intake to 6-10 a day.

Tendinitis

Description:

Tendinitis occurs when the cords attaching bone to muscle are inflamed, resulting in pain and strain. This can be caused by repeated stress being placed on the specified tendon and causing tearing. Tendonitis often occurs in the hips, wrists, knees, shoulders, elbows, ankles, or heels.

Application:

Dilute your chosen oil accordingly (2-3 drops Soothing Blend or Birch coupled with Lemongrass is suggested) with a carrier oil and massage into the affected area 2-3 times daily. A few minutes following application layer with Peppermint.

Recommended Oils:

Wintergreen, Soothing Blend, Rosemary, Peppermint, Massage Blend, Marjoram, Oregano, Lemongrass, Lemon, Lavender, Helichrysum, Eucalyptus, Cypress, Birch, and Basil

Other Natural Protocols:

Ginger helps reduce inflammation. Combine equal parts Ginger juice, Honey, and Pomegranate juice in a glass jug and consume one tablespoon 2-3 times daily.

Chapter 3:
Brain Health

The body's control center is composed of the brain and nervous system, which dictate the body's movements, stores thoughts and memories, analyzes the senses, and helps regulate other bodily systems and organs. The brain sends signals to the body through nerves, which are pathways that run to every point of the body; for instance, your spinal cord is a nerve pathway that extends from your brain right down through the middle of your back.

Aging produces changes in the brain and nervous system, such as atrophy, in which nerve cells are lost. The nerve cells also decrease, meaning the messages passed from the brain to the rest of the body may be transmitted at a slower rate. Moreover, nerve cells begin to break down in the brain tissue, creating waste products that may produce abnormalities in the brain, such as plaques or lipofuscin.

Such breakdowns in the nerve cells can impact senses, which reduce sensations and reflexes, as well as the senses of sight, smell, and taste. Memory, cognitive processing, and thought may also slow with age due to these changes in the brain and nervous system.

Anti-aging Brain & Nervous System Care 101: Essential Oils & Preventative Protocols

Just as with the rest of the body, the brain needs healthy diet and exercise to combat aging. Neurodegeneration is a natural result of aging, but it can occur with less severity and at a slower rate when preventative protocols are regularly exercised.

To maintain the health of your brain and nervous system consider both physical and mental exercise. Physical exercise will pump a sufficient amount of blood to the brain, which reduces the loss of brain cells, while mental exercise – like doing word puzzles, reading, debating, or participating in regular intellectual discussions, etc. – will keep your mind as sharp as a tack.

There are also "superfoods" that promote brain function, many of which double to promote skin health. These include nuts and seeds, avocados, salmon (or other fish high in omega-3s), whole grains, blueberries, tomatoes, broccoli, and sage.

The antioxidant properties of essential oils can support

your anti-aging efforts when it comes to the brain and nervous system. Consider the following study, published by *Journal of Oleo Science*, in which the antioxidant effects of Lemon essential oil on neurodegeneration were examined.

Study 4 – Antioxidant Properties

"This study sought to investigate the effects of essential oil from Lemon (Citrus limon) peels on acetylcholinesterase (AChE) and butyrylcholinesterase (BChE) activities in vitro... The inhibition of AChE and BChE activities, inhibition of pro-oxidant induced lipid peroxidation and antioxidant activities could be possible mechanisms for the use of the essential oil in the management and prevention of oxidative stress-induced neurodegeneration."

By testing Lemon essential oil against acetylcholinesterase and butyrylcholinesterase, both of which are enzymes which actively terminate neurotransmission, the study found that Lemon essential oil inhibits the damaging activity of these enzymes. This, alongside the oil's antioxidant properties, means that Lemon essential oil may have the potential to support the body's natural defenses against neurodegenerative diseases, such as Alzheimer's, ALS, Huntington's, or Parkinson's.

Reference:
http://www.ncbi.nlm.nih.gov/pubmed/24599102]

https://www.jstage.jst.go.jp/article/jos/63/4/63_ess13166
/_pdf]

Along with diet and exercise the following essential oil protocols can support healthy brain and nervous system function; priming your brain to combat the effects of aging.

Essential Oil Protocols

Brain Function

Description:

The following protocols can help promote optimum brain function and mental clarity.

Application:

• General health – dilute your essential oil accordingly (Grounding Blend, Melissa, or Frankincense are suggested) and apply topically to the brain stem and the soles of the feet.

Recommended Oils:

Ylang Ylang, Sandalwood, Rosemary, Peppermint, Patchouli, Oregano, Myrrh, Melissa, Marjoram, Lavender, Helichrysum, Frankincense, Grounding Blend, Cypress,

Clove, Cinnamon, Cassia, Calming Blend, and Basil

Other Natural Protocols:

Consider essential oil-based products, like Basic Vitality Supplements (LLV). Coconut oil can also improve cognitive performance and help with brain issues, as it influences amyloid-β (Aβ), a component that contributes to degeneration. Twice a day, eat 1-2 teaspoons of organic, cold-pressed, non-hydrogenated, virgin coconut oil.

Circulation

Description:

Poor circulation is when blood flows insufficiently, which is particularly noticeable in the feet, legs, and hands, where cramping or fatigue may occur. Poor circulation may become chronic and can lead to varicose veins, kidney issues, open ulcers, stroke, and slow healing. Proper circulation can also promote brain function.

Application:

For immediate relief, dilute your chosen essential oil accordingly (Cypress, Massage Blend, Coriander, Lemongrass, and Protective Blend are suggested) and apply topically to the affected area. You can also blend Frankincense, Lemongrass, Cypress, and Marjoram in equal parts, diluted with a carrier oil, and apply the blend to the soles of the feet and the heart.

Recommended Oils:

Ylang Ylang, Sandalwood, Protective Blend, Peppermint, Myrrh, Massage Blend, Marjoram, Lemongrass, Lemon, Invigorating Blend, Ginger, Geranium, Frankincense, Eucalyptus, Cypress, Coriander, Black Pepper, and Basil

Other Natural Protocols:

Also consider essential oil-based products, like the Basic Vitality Supplements (LLV), which will assist with long-term care of this issue. Garlic's active ingredient, allicin, helps improve blood flow. For the best results, eat 3-4 Cloves of garlic a day on an empty stomach.

Common Brain-Aging Issues & Essential Oil Protocols

Normal aging processes do not involve severe dementia or memory loss, but these are the side effects of some common neurodegenerative diseases, like Alzheimer's. Such conditions occur as a result of the buildup of lipofuscin, which causes plaques in the brain.

Other health conditions that can contribute to neurodegeneration include diabetes, infection, and the consumption of certain medications, which may cause delirium and severe confusion in the elderly. Such issues are often not directly related to the brain, but rather to the illnesses. Diabetes, in particular, interferes with mental cognition when the blood sugar levels rise and fall erratically.

If you are faced with changes in thinking, behavior, or memory which stray from normal patterns or interfere with day-to-day tasks, seek advice from a healthcare provider to help diagnose the cause, then support the cause with the below essential oil protocols.

Essential Oil Protocols

Alzheimer's Disease

Description:

Alzheimer's disease leads to dementia and includes mood swings, changes in social behavior, memory loss, as well as the loss of other brain functions which influence language skills, judgement, and social skills. Alzheimer's is believed to be influenced by genetics, head injuries, prolonged high blood pressure, aging and recent studies show, nutritional deficiencies. The disease is progressive and will cause brain cells to degenerate, steadily enhancing the symptoms, which also include slowness, difficulty in multitasking, violent or unusual behavior, losing things, disinterest, a change in sleep patterns, and an inability to understand situations around them.

Application:

• Cognitive impairment – dilute your essential oil accordingly (Patchouli is suggested) and apply topically to the brain stem and the soles of the feet. You may also apply a drop under the tongue.

• General health – dilute your essential oil accordingly (Grounding Blend, Melissa, or Frankincense are suggested) and apply topically to the brain stem and the soles of the feet.

Recommended Oils:

Ylang Ylang, Sandalwood, Rosemary, Peppermint, Patchouli, Oregano, Myrrh, Melissa, Marjoram, Lavender, Helichrysum, Frankincense, Grounding Blend, Cypress, Clove, Cinnamon, Cassia, Calming Blend, and Basil

Other Natural Protocols:

Consider essential oil-based products, like Basic Vitality Supplements (LLV). Coconut oil can also improve cognitive performance and help with brain issues, as it influences amyloid-β (Aβ), one of the disease's components. Twice a day, eat 1-2 teaspoons of organic, cold-pressed, non-hydrogenated, virgin coconut oil only. Ginkgo biloba also helps alleviate anxiety, as well as improve memory and cognitive function. Every day, take a standard 120-mg capsule daily divided into 2-3 doses.

Dementia

Description:

Dementia describes a group of symptoms that are common in a great many diseases, including loss of judgement, memory, social skills, language skills, and other brain functions. Dementia is the result of advanced age and diseases, like multiple sclerosis, Huntington's, Parkinson's, or diseases associated with aging, like Alzheimer's. Other issues that may contribute to dementia include alcoholism, nutritional deficiencies, brain infection, and tumors.

Application:

Basic care – dilute your chosen oil accordingly (Frankincense, Melissa, and Grounding Blend are suggested) with a carrier oil and apply topically to the back of the neck along the brainstem two times a day.

Recommended Oils:

Ylang Ylang, Sandalwood, Rosemary, Peppermint, Patchouli, Oregano, Myrrh, Melissa, Marjoram, Lavender, Helichrysum, Grounding Blend, Geranium, Frankincense, Cypress, Clove, Cinnamon, Cassia, Calming Blend, and Basil

Other Natural Protocols:

Consider essential oil-based products, like Basic Vitality Supplements (LLV). Ginkgo biloba helps alleviate anxiety, as well as improve memory and cognitive function.

Every day take a standard 120-mg capsule divided into 2-3 doses.

Diabetes

Description:

Diabetes is a condition that occurs when glucose cannot be delivered to cells in the blood stream. Glucose is sugar broken down from our food that, once broken down works as fuel for fat, muscle, and liver cells. The pancreas provides insulin, which helps assimilate the glucose and so, when not enough insulin is produced, glucose is not assimilated, leading to high blood sugar. Symptoms of diabetes include blurred eyesight, weight loss, increased thirst, and urination, fatigue, numbness and tingling of feet. Three types of diabetes exist: Type 1 (juvenile diabetes), Type 2 (most common form, often associated with aging, family history and physical inactivity), and Gestational Diabetes (occurs during pregnancy).

Application:

Type 2 – for topical application, massage Grounding Blend into the feet in the morning and Lavender at night. For internal application, place 8-10 drops of your chosen oil (Basil and Coriander are suggested; add 2 drops of Protective Blend for added support) into a capsule and take daily.

Recommended Oils:

Protective Blend, Peppermint, Marjoram, Lavender, Helichrysum, Grounding Blend, Geranium, Frankincense, Eucalyptus, Cypress, Coriander, Clove, Cinnamon, Cassia, and Basil

Other Natural Protocols:

Consider essential oil-based products, like Basic Vitality Supplements (LLV), Digestive Enzyme Complex, GI Cleansing Formula/Probiotic Defense Formula, and ongoing Detoxification Blend. Support proper nutrition and weight management with regular diet and exercise. Bitter gourd influences the glucose metabolism, aiding in pancreatic insulin secretion. Each morning remove the seeds from 2-3 bitter gourds, juice the fruits, add the juice to water, and drink the bitter gourd juice before eating.

Nerve Damage

Description:

Nerve damage may be caused by a number of diseases, such as autoimmune disease, IBD, multiple sclerosis, diabetes, ALS, or lupus. It can also be caused by infections (Lyme, Hepatitis, HIV), cancer growths, cancer treatments, medicine, drugs, toxins, arthritic pressure, trauma, or a myriad of other issues. As a result, symptoms vary according to cause, but they may include sensory damage (dizziness, pain, tingling, numbness, burning), motor damage (paralysis, weakness, twitching, muscle atrophy), and autoimmune damage (constipation, dry mouth, dry eyes, sexual dysfunction, bladder issues, and excessive perspiration).

Application:

To restore damaged nerves, manage pain, boost circulation, and protect against infection, combine 15 drops Geranium, 10 drops each Wintergreen and Helichrysum, 8 drops Marjoram, 6 drops Cypress, 5 drops Peppermint, and 2 drops each Lemon and Clove in a small glass bottle or container. Blend well, dilute 3-4 drops with a carrier oil, and apply topically to affected area up to three times daily.

Recommended Oils:

Vetiver, Roman Chamomile, Peppermint, Patchouli, Massage Blend, Marjoram, Oregano, Lemongrass, Lemon, Lavender, Juniper, Helichrysum, Grounding Blend,

Grapefruit, Geranium, Cypress, Cassia, and Birch

Other Natural Protocols:

Apply a warm compress to the affected area for 5-7 minutes to relieve numbness and discomfort.

Neuropathy

Description:

Neuropathy (or peripheral neuropathy) occurs when the peripheral nervous system is damaged, due to infection, toxins, malnutrition, trauma, or certain diseases like diabetes. Peripheral neuropathy can take many forms, such as carpal tunnel syndrome, and commonly involves the loss of sensation, loss of muscle control, numbness, tingling, or burning.

Application:

For neuropathy of the feet, massage 2-4 drops Grounding Blend into the feet, then blend 2-4 drops each of Marjoram, Cypress, and Basil and massage into the feet. Top with 2-4 drops Peppermint, then apply a hot compress.

See other protocols per underlying conditions.

Recommended Oils:

Peppermint, Marjoram, Grounding Blend, Cypress, and Basil

Other Natural Protocols:

Take a 100 milligram supplement of vitamin B-1 every day. Also apply cayenne cream to affected area to relieve neuropathy pain.

Parkinson's Disease

Description:

Parkinson's disease is a common nervous system disorder that occurs due to an insufficient amount of dopamine reaching the area of the brain that coordinates body movements, resulting in tremors, shaking, and difficulties with walking. Parkinson's is a progressive disease and often affects elderly folks over the age of 50. Early symptoms include trembling, a feeling of limpness, and lack of facial expression, while advanced symptoms include constipation, drooling, difficulty with mobility, increased trembling, muscle pain, depression, dementia, and anxiety.

Application:

For internal application, place 1-2 drops Frankincense under the tongue. Topically apply Frankincense to the crown of the head, the base of the skull, and the spine. Additionally, dilute your chosen oil accordingly (Wild Orange, Tea Tree, Grounding Blend, Protective Blend, Lavender, Peppermint, Massage Blend, or Soothing Blend are suggested) with a carrier oil and, using the Massage Blend technique, apply topically.

Recommended Oils:

Ylang Ylang, Wild Orange, Peppermint, Myrrh, Lavender, Grounding Blend, Ginger, Frankincense, Cypress, and Basil

Other Natural Protocols:

Consider essential oil-based products, like Basic Vitality Supplements (LLV), GI Cleansing Formula, and Probiotic Defense Formula. To support mental acuity, always maintain a healthy diet and eating habits. Fish oil is rich in omega-3 fatty acids and can help stimulate hormone production, nerve tissue health, and brain functionality. For the proper dosage on fish oil supplements, consult your doctor.

Stroke

Description:

Strokes occur when any part of the brain does not receive its proper supply of blood, due to blood vessel blockage or brain bleeding, which results in brain cell death in a matter of minutes. Symptoms include double vision, trouble speaking, headache, confusion, difficulty walking, lack of balance, numbness, paralysis, or tingling in one side of the body, particularly in the arm or the face. Strokes can be hemorrhagic (damage to a brain's blood vessel), ischemic (blockage in the blood supply), or transient ischemic attack (mini-stroke; blood is blocked briefly but then resumes).

Application:

General recovery – after seeking medical attention follow an internal application protocol of 1-2 drops Frankincense under the tongue 2-5 times each day. Couple this with a topical application of Massage Blend over the area of the heart.

Recommended Oils:

Ylang Ylang, Peppermint, Melissa, Massage Blend, Lavender, Helichrysum, Grounding Blend, Grapefruit, Frankincense, Cypress, and Basil

Other Natural Protocols:

Consider essential oil-based products, like Basic Vitality Supplements (LLV). In the case of a stroke, always seek immediate medical attention. To reduce risk of stroke, live a healthy lifestyle – meaning eat healthy, exercise, limit alcohol consumption, do not smoke, regulate your blood pressure, and manage stress.*Prior to each meal, apply 1-2 drops to your drinking water.*

Chapter 4:
Sensory Function (Vision, Hearing, Taste, Smell, & Touch)

Our senses receive information from the environment, and this information – light, sound, smell, taste, and touch – is delivered in the form of nerve signals to the brain, which then interprets these sensations.

With age comes wisdom; but the physiological fact is that with age you truly do see the world differently because your senses change. The way you see, hear, taste, touch, and smell dulls as the years pass away. Such changes can impact quality of life, in that activities become less enjoyable, communication becomes more difficult, and the individual may begin to feel isolated. As the information received from the environment becomes less sharp, the minimum level of stimulation required to absorb any sensation (called the threshold) increases; this means that the threshold becomes greater as we age.

Although sight and hearing are often the most affected by aging, all senses can be impacted. Equipment and other devices are regularly introduced to improve the senses and quality of life for the elderly (hearing aids and glasses, for example), but other efforts can be made to prevent sensory aging, or support these natural changes. Let's take a look at each of the senses, in turn, and the protocols that can help.

Vision

Light is processed by the eye as it passes through the cornea, continues through the pupil, and is interpreted by the brain. This is why the pupil shrinks and expands – it is controlling the amount of light that enters the eye. Once the light enters, the lens of the inner eye refocuses the light on the retina, converting the light into nerve signals which are sent to the brain by the optic nerve.

As we age, the pupils reduce in size; in fact, they shrink by around 2/3 from the ages of 20 - 60. They also react differently to bright light and darkness and the cornea becomes less sensitive, making injuries to the eye less noticeable. Moreover, the lens of the eye clouds, yellows, and becomes less flexible, while the eye muscles rotate less freely. Floaters also may obstruct your vision. With age these particles, called vitreous float in the eye and although not blinding, they can be irritating. Weakened eye muscles limit peripheral vision, causing field of vision to narrow. All of this contributes to the decline of vision, with focusing becoming more difficult, glare less tolerable, and adeptness at seeing in the dark reduced significantly. This makes driving at night, or being outside in the bright light of afternoon, hard on the eyes.

It also becomes more difficult to differentiate between cool colors, like blues and greens. This is why warm and contrasting colors can improve vision and it's even recommended to light the hallways at night with a red light rather than a white one.

Additionally, aging eyes produce less tears, leading to dry eyes, which are more susceptible to inflammation, infection, and scarring of the cornea. Eye disorders, like macular degeneration, glaucoma, or cataracts can also occur.

Eye exercises may help to improve vision due to eyestrain, increased sensitivity to light, and blurred vision. By building up the muscles in the eyes, focus and eye movements are improved. The brain's vision center is also stimulated through progressive exercises that help control eye muscle movements. Some examples include covering each eye in turn, and focusing on different objects, or concentrating focus on one object, or following a visual pattern. These natural protocols vary according to the patient's existing eye problem and their age.

Essential oils can help with macular degeneration. Consider this study, published by *Molecular Vision*, which examined the effects of a combination of zinc oxide and Rosemary oil on light-induced oxidative retinal damage.

Study 5 - Vision

"Zinc oxide effectively reduces visual cell loss in rats exposed to intense visible light and is known to slow the rate of disease progression in advanced stages of age-related macular degeneration. Our goal was to determine the efficacy of zinc oxide in combination with novel and well-established antioxidants in an animal model of light-induced oxidative retinal damage...In the rat model of acute retinal light damage, zinc oxide combined with a detergent extract of Rosemary powder or Rosemary oil is more effective than treatment with either component alone and significantly more effective than an AREDS mixture containing a comparable dose of zinc oxide. Light-induced oxidative stress in animal models of retinal degeneration can be a useful preclinical paradigm for screening novel antioxidants and for testing potential therapeutics designed to slow the progression of age-related ocular disease."

In the study one group of rats was treated with zinc oxide, or Rosemary extract separately, after which they were exposed to intense light for 4-24 hours. A second group received a combination of zinc oxide and Rosemary oil, while a third group received an antioxidant mineral mix containing zinc oxide. After two weeks' intensive light treatment the visual cell survival of the rats was determined, and the results indicated that the Rosemary-zinc combination promoted visual cell survival and reduced the expression of oxidative stress protein markers. This suggests that essential oils – particularly Rosemary – may be effective supplements in visual therapy treatments and can protect against macular degeneration and disease.

Reference
http://www.ncbi.nlm.nih.gov/pubmed/23825923]

http://www.ncbi.nlm.nih.gov/pmc/articles/PMC3695758/
pdf/mv-v19-1433.pdf]

Essential Oil Protocols

Loss of Eyesight

Description:

Presbyopia (failing eyesight) occurs naturally with aging as the elasticity of the eye's lens is lost. Different forms of presbyopia include cataracts – cloudy or foggy vision, resulting from diseases like diabetes, eye surgery, trauma, congenital defect, or radiation –, glaucoma –, drainage of eye fluid is impeded and causes damage in the optic nerve; may cause loss of sight –, retinal detachment –, distortion of vision caused by the retina separating from the underlying tissue; may be the result of trauma, inflammatory disorders, and diseases like diabetes –, uveitis/irititis – inflammation or irritation of the iris or uvea, caused by autoimmune disorders or infection –, and macular degeneration – blur of the central zone of vision, resulting from aging.

Application:

For regeneration, place 1-2 drops of your chosen oil on your fingertip (Anti-Aging Blend, Frankincense, and Helichrysum are suggested) and dab the oil around the eye socket but not in the eye. Do this up to three times daily. Also, dilute your chosen oil with a carrier oil and massage into the reflex points of the feet. Those eye problems that stem from infection (like uveitis and iritis) can benefit from a Detoxification Cleanse or from an Anti-infectant protocol.

Recommended Oils:

Ylang Ylang, Sandalwood, Rosemary, Lemongrass, Lavender, Helichrysum, Frankincense, Cypress, and Anti-Aging Blend

Other Natural Protocols:

Consider essential oil-based products, like the Detoxification Blend, the GI Cleansing Formula, and the Probiotic Defense Formula. Ginkgo biloba improves circulation in the eye, protecting against issues of macular degeneration and glaucoma, while improving vision. Every day take a standard 120-mg capsule divided into 2-3 doses.

Hearing

The ears are double-functional: they maintain the body's balance and of course, they hear. Balance is controlled by the small hairs and fluid in the inner ear, which are transmitted via the auditory nerve to the brain, thereby assisting in maintaining equilibrium. Hearing occurs when sound vibrations enter the inner ear through the eardrum, after which the inner ear transmits the vibrations into nerve signals which are then sent to the brain via the auditory nerve.

Aging changes the structures of the inner ear, resulting in declining function and reducing the ear's capacity to decipher sound and maintain balance. Hearing loss often affects both ears and is particularly relevant when it comes to high-frequency sounds and differentiating between particular sounds. Background noise may also influence your ability to hear, while other conditions – like tinnitus – may produce abnormal noises, like ringing. These issues can be due to aging or earwax buildup.

Essential Oil Protocols

Hearing Loss

Description:

Loss of hearing occurs when one or both ears can no longer hear at normal levels and as a result, may not be able to comprehend certain words, frequencies, or when there is background noise. Hearing loss happens naturally with age and can include conductive hearing loss (eardrum damage due to wax buildup, fluids, injury, or infection), sensorineural hearing loss (nerve endings inside the ear aren't responding correctly due to age, disease, or medication), and congenital hearing loss (hearing impairments at birth due to genetic defect or infection).

Application:

Blend 4 drops each of Calming Blend and Grounding Blend. Apply topically to the front of the ear over the fleshy rim, down the earlobe, and down the Eustachian tubes under and behind the ears and behind the jaw line. Repeat 10 times. Apply 4 drops Helichrysum in the same method and repeat 5 times. Blend 2 drops each of White Fir and Lavender and apply in the same method. Repeat 5 times. Apply 3 drops Geranium in the same method and repeat 3 times. Cup and inhale. Repeat this protocol 2-3 times weekly for 6-8 weeks.

Recommended Oils:

White Fir, Lavender, Helichrysum, Geranium, Fennel, Eucalyptus, Grounding Blend, and Calming Blend

Other Natural Protocols:

Ginkgo biloba improves blood circulation and can help with hearing loss. Every day take a standard 120-mg capsule divided into 2-3 doses.

Tinnitus

Description:

Tinnitus occurs when a disruptive sound (ringing, whistling, clicking, buzzing, crickets) is heard in the ears, with either mild or intolerable results. Tinnitus is a symptom which often indicates an underlying health issue, such as ear infection, allergy fluids, physical damage to the eardrum (loud noises), or wax buildup. It can also be caused by aging or certain medications.

Application:

Blend 1 drop each of Basil and Frankincense and apply topically behind the ear and down the jaw line to the chin. Repeat several times and follow the protocol every 1-4 hours, or until the sound ceases.

Recommended Oils:

Rosemary, Peppermint, Lavender, Helichrysum, Geranium, Frankincense, Cypress, and Basil

Other Natural Protocols:

Consider essential oil-based products, like GI Cleansing Formula or Probiotic Defense Formula. Ginkgo biloba improves blood circulation and can help with hearing loss. Every day take a standard 120-mg capsule divided into 2-3 doses.

Vertigo

Description:

Vertigo occurs when the body is imbalanced often due to a disconnection between the inner ear's vestibular organ and the brain. Vertigo makes your surroundings seem as though they are in motion, which creates unbalance and nausea. The issue may also be due to physical trauma, inflammation, or chemical issues.

Application:

To protect against vertigo, dilute your chosen oil accordingly (Ginger is suggested) with a carrier oil and apply topically to the affected area. You can also place a few drops in a capsule and take orally. To relieve an attack, place a couple drops of your chosen oil (Frankincense is suggested) under the tongue when feelings of instability come upon you. Repeat after 30 minutes.

Recommended Oils:

Ylang Ylang, Thyme, Rosemary, Roman Chamomile, Peppermint, Lavender, Helichrysum, Ginger, Geranium, Frankincense, and Basil

Other Natural Protocols:

Consider essential oil-based products, like the Basic Vitality Supplement (LLV). If you are feeling dizzy, then try deep breathing to relax the nervous system and provide oxygen to the brain: lie down or sit down comfortably, place one hand on the abdomen and the thumb of the other hand against one nostril, close the mouth, inhale slowly until the lungs are full of air, hold the breath for 2-3 seconds, then exhale slowly. Repeat 10 times and sit calmly for 5 minutes until dizziness passes.

Taste and Smell

Taste and smell are symbiotic senses as odors often directly contribute to the sense of taste. The nerve endings in the lining of the upper nose are where smell begins, while taste is determined by the nearly 9,000 taste buds which decipher between salty, sweet, bitter, and sour tastes. Together they serve to identify dangers, such as gases, smoke, decay, or spoilage.

As you age taste buds reduce in amount, they lose mass and their ability to decipher between the four tastes declines. Moreover, less saliva is being produced, which can result in dry mouth. This may also influence taste.

Smell may decline as well due to the nose's loss of nerve endings coupled with less mucus being produced. With this lack of nerve endings and reduction in mucus odors are not held in the nose long enough to be identified. Nasal polyps may also be interfering with smell and may even cause breathing problems.

Some factors that influence the rate at which you lose these senses include smoking, certain diseases, and exposure to pollution and other destructive air particles. When taste and smell are lost, the risk of danger increases, as the sense of smell often triggers our attention to harmful situations, such as fire or poisonous gases. Additionally, appetite may be reduced, as without working taste buds, there is no longer any enjoyment gleaned from eating.

There are some natural protocols that may help with the loss of taste and smell. These include altering your food preparation to include certain spices that trigger taste, like Ginger or garlic. You might also consider talking to your healthcare provider if issues are due to a particular medication you have been prescribed.

Essential oils can help stimulate taste and smell in the following ways.

Essential Oil Protocols

Dry Mouth

Description:

Dry mouth and bad breath (halitosis) are often caused by health issues, poor oral hygiene, or aging. Unhealthy lifestyle habits can exacerbate the issue, as can the foods you eat.

Application:

Apply two drops of your chosen oil to your tongue.

Recommended Oils:

Wintergreen, Peppermint, Fennel, and Digestive Blend

Other Natural Protocols:

Consider essential oil-based products, like Peppermint Beadlets. Fennel can also eliminate dry mouth and bad breath, so chew a tablespoon of Fennel seeds slowly as it will stimulate saliva production.

Loss of Smell (Anosmia)

Description:

Loss of smell, or anosmia, is either a temporary or long-term condition whereby the physical passageways from the nasal passages to the olfactory cells are obstructed or the nerve passages in the brain are not properly functioning. Loss of smell can affect taste since the two are connected. Causes of anosmia include sinus congestion, allergies, nasal polyps, toxic chemicals, medications, drugs, nutritional/hormonal imbalance, and some diseases, such as Parkinson's, Alzheimer's, or multiple sclerosis.

Application:

• Clear nasal obstructions – diffuse or use the cupping method to inhale the Respiratory Blend. Or dilute your chosen essential oil accordingly (Rosemary, Basil, and Tea Tree are suggested) and apply to the sinuses, over the nose and eyebrows.

• Stimulate olfactory – inhale Respiratory Blend or Peppermint directly and frequently using the cupping method.

Recommended Oils:

Rosemary, Respiratory Blend, Peppermint, Tea Tree, Lime, and Basil

Other Natural Protocols:

Consider GI Cleansing Formula/Probiotic Defense Formula or Cellular Complex. Warm a tbsp. of castor oil in the microwave for a few seconds and place one drop in each nostril twice a day, morning and night.

Nasal Polyps

Description:

A polyp is a mostly benign, but sometimes precancerous or cancerous protuberance of tissue from a mucus membrane, which may be directly attached or have a long stock connecting it to the body. They commonly occur on the colon, the cervix, nasal passages, and the urinary bladder. Symptoms include abnormal bleeding (cervical polyps) or breathing problems (nasal polyps).

Application:

Nasal polyp – place 1-3 drops of your chosen oil (Frankincense or Tea Tree are suggested) on a Q-tip and apply to the bridge of the nose and beneath the tongue. You can also take internally in a capsule up to twice a day.

Other polyps – place 1-3 drops Frankincense under the tongue or take internally in a capsule.

Recommended Oils:

Peppermint, Oregano, Tea Tree, Lemon, Lavender, Grounding Blend, Frankincense, Cleansing Blend, and Basil

Other Natural Protocols:

Get rid of toxins by eating cayenne pepper or drinking hot tea in heat. Either will induce sweating, ridding the body of toxins that sometimes influence polyp growth.

Touch (Pain & Vibration)

Touch involves the nerve endings in tendons, joints, muscles, skin, and internal organs sending information to the brain about temperature, vibration, pressure, pain, and the position of the body. While often this information may be subconscious, other times the information may cause acute sensation, as the brain identifies the type and intensity of touch.

As you age these sensations may alter or decrease due to nerve ending damage, decreased blood flow, or brain/spinal cord injury. Being as such, many of the applications associated with the brain – such as <u>circulation</u> and <u>nerve damage</u> – can also support the loss of this sense. Health issues, as well, can cause alterations in sensation, as can a lack of nutrients.

When the ability to sense touch is reduced, then there is an increased risk of injury due to temperature, especially in regards to burns, hypothermia, or frostbite. The individual may also be oblivious to pressure ulcers, other pain, or injuries due to this reduction in sensitivity. On the opposite end of the spectrum, some individuals develop abnormal sensitivity to a light touch of the skin due to the thinning of aging skin.

Some protocols to stay safe include dressing for the weather, noting the temperature of hot water to prevent burns, and inspecting oneself for injury.

Essential Oil Protocols

Heat Exhaustion/Heat Stroke

Description:

Heat exhaustion occurs when the body's ability to cool itself is inadequate to the physical exertion, due to extremely hot or humid climates, dehydration, or sweating. Symptoms include an increase in temperature, flushed face, weakness, and disorientation. Heat stroke occurs if the temperature rises above 104 F. Seek medical attention, as symptoms of heat stroke also include increased heart rate, vomiting, diarrhea, convulsions/seizures, unconsciousness, and flushed color in other body parts.

Application:

Add a couple drops of Peppermint to a cool, damp cloth and apply to the forehead. For topical application, apply 2-3 drops of Peppermint to the chest, the neck, the back of the neck, and the soles of the feet. Use the cup and inhale method and if the body temperature rises extremely give the patient a sponge bath.

Recommended Oils:

Peppermint and Lavender

Other Natural Protocols:

First and foremost, always move the person to a shady and cool area, rehydrate them with cool beverages (avoid carbonated drinks and alcohol), and place them in a restful position.

Sensory Processing Disorder

Description:

Sensory Processing Disorder (SPD) occurs when information from the senses is not being processed correctly, resulting in overreactions or under reactions to certain sensory experiences, like sensitivity to light, touch, certain textures, odors, or demonstrations of unusual distress and fear, tantrums over minor events, ignoring or not interacting with others, appearing uncoordinated, or requiring sensory stimulus before being able to sleep. The reason for this disorder is unknown.

Application:

Dilute chosen oil accordingly (a blend of 18 drops Vetiver, 10 drops Lavender, 10 drops Ylang Ylang, 7 drops Frankincense, 5 drops Clary Sage, 3 drops Marjoram and 12 drops fractionated coconut oil in a roller bottle is suggested; use only a roll of the blend) with a carrier oil and apply topically to the soles of the feet, the back of the neck, and the suboccipital triangle.

*note: do not force odors or massage onto individuals with SPD, as they are sometimes sensitive to these things. Allow them to select their own oil scent.

Recommended Oils:

Ylang Ylang, Vetiver, Marjoram, Lavender, Frankincense, and Clary Sage

Chapter 5:
Blend Recipes for Essential Oils & Aging

In this chapter, we will provide various recipes for blends of essential oils that promote anti-aging, or support aging conditions. Herbalists and aromatherapists often recommend combining several essential oils that complement each other to effectively utilize the best properties of each and to produce the best possible results.

Safety Precautions

Safety Singles

Certain adverse effects may evolve when using pure essential oils. Some essential oils should not be used when pregnant for example, as they may cause miscarriage. Allergic reactions may occur, especially when applied topically. Always administer an allergy test before committing fully to topical application. When used with other medications essential oils may react negatively. If you are on any current prescription medications or have a chronic illness, such as high blood pressure, epilepsy, or liver disease, then researching the effects of essential oils against your own personal medical history will eliminate any potentially problematic issues.

Blends

Oftentimes essential oils are manufactured as blends of several pure oils. For instance, the Protective Blend of certain brands is a mix of Cinnamon, Clove, Rosemary, and Eucalyptus. This blend can be used to boost the immune system to help support colds, viruses, and flus. The downside to blends is that the more oils added to the mix, the higher the probability the patient may react negatively to the blend if he/she is prone to allergies. There is also the possibility of photo toxicity when working with blends, particularly if they include citrus oils. Be sure to read your labels before administering.

Blends

Anti-Aging Salve

Ingredients

5 drops Geranium Essential Oil

5 drops Frankincense Essential Oil

5 drops Myrrh Essential Oil

5 drops Rosemary Essential Oil

5 drops Lemon Essential Oil

10 drops Rosehip Essential Oil

10 drops Carrot Seed Essential Oil

10 drops Sandalwood Essential Oil

½ cup Apricot Kernel Oil

Directions

To reduce the signs of skin aging combine all ingredients in a small glass jar or container, blending well. After your evening facial routine apply to areas of concern. Use as needed, blending well before each use.

Arthritic Massage Oil

Ingredients

2 drops Black Pepper Essential Oil

2 drops Ginger Essential Oil

3 drops Coriander Essential Oil

4 drops Helichrysum Essential Oil

5 drops Roman Chamomile Essential Oil

2 ounces Carrier Oil

Directions

To relieve arthritic pain, combine all ingredients in a small bowl, blending well. Apply topically, massaging the oil into the affected area. Use as needed.

Blood Sugar

Ingredients

8 drops Cinnamon Essential Oil

8 drops Clove Essential Oil

10 drops Thyme Essential Oil

15 drops Rosemary Essential Oil

2 ounces V-6

Directions

To help maintain insulin levels, combine all ingredients and apply topically to feet and over pancreas.

Brain Stimulant

Ingredients

30 drops Balsam Fir Essential Oil

15 drops Sandalwood Essential Oil

15 drops Frankincense Essential Oil

8 drops Helichrysum Essential oil

3 drops Melissa Essential Oil

2 drops Peppermint Essential Oil

1-ounce Carrier Oil

Directions

To help stimulate the brain combine all ingredients in a small glass bottle or container and blend well. When needed apply 10-12 drops of the blend per ounce of carrier oil and massage into the temples, forehead, back of the neck, and into the reflex points of the feet.

Citrus Oil Detoxifier

Ingredients

1 drop Tangerine Essential Oil

1 drops Lemon Essential Oil

1 drop Grapefruit Essential Oil

24 ounces Water (separated)

Directions

Drinking plenty of water throughout the day is not only a good way to stay hydrated and healthy, but it also flushes out toxins, which interfere with hormonal balance. Citrus oils are particularly beneficial to cleansing the body (particularly the lymphatic system) of these toxins. Add a single drop of one of the oils to each 8 ounces of drinking water throughout the day to reduce toxins, aid hormone balance, and increase libido.

Stress Bath

Ingredients

2 drops Rosemary Essential Oil

3 drops Black Pepper Essential Oil

5 drops Grapefruit Essential Oil

1 Tbsp. Grapeseed Oil

Directions

To wind down, de-stress, and combat anxiety, add all ingredients to your bathwater and stir to disperse. Then inhale deeply while you soak for 20 minutes, but avoid getting water in your eyes as it may sting.

Detoxifying Bath

Ingredients

2 drops Juniper Berry Essential Oil

2 drops Geranium Essential Oil

2 drops Lavender Essential Oil

2 drops Rosemary Essential Oil

Directions

For a bath that detoxes the body's systems add all ingredients to your bathwater and stir to disperse. Inhale deeply while you soak for 20 minutes, but avoid getting water in your eyes as it may sting.

142

Detoxifying Blend

Ingredients

2 drops Juniper Berry Essential Oil

2 drops Lavender Essential Oil

2 drops Grapefruit Essential Oil

2 drops Basil Essential Oil

2 drops Cypress Essential Oil

30 mL Carrier Oil

Directions

To flush out toxins and boost circulation combine all ingredients, blending well, and massage into the reflex points in the feet.

Energy Booster

Ingredients

10 drops Orange Essential Oil

10 drops Cinnamon Essential Oil

10 drops Black Pepper Essential Oil

Directions

Diffuse blend throughout your home to stimulate energy.

Fatigue

Ingredients

4 drops Rosemary Essential Oil

2 drops Basil Essential Oil

30 mL Carrier Oil

Directions

To combat exhaustion combine all ingredients, blending well, and massage into the reflex points in the feet.

Hand Nourishing Cream

Ingredients

2 drops Rose Essential Oil

2 drops Melissa Essential Oil

2 drops Roman Chamomile Essential Oil

15 grams Cocoa Butter

7 grams Beeswax

30 mL Orange Flower Water

20 mL Avocado Oil

20 mL PrimRose Carrier Oil

5 mL Carrot Seed Essential Oil

Directions

To nourish and moisturize the hands mix all ingredients in a small glass jar or container until well combined and apply topically as needed, massaging the cream into the hands, nails, and cuticles.

Harmonious Diffusion Blend

Ingredients

   1 drops Grapefruit Essential Oil

   1 drop Ylang Ylang Essential Oil

   1 drop Wild Orange Essential Oil

   2 drops Patchouli Essential Oil

   3 drops Bergamot Essential Oil

Directions

   To support harmony in a tense home or mind, combine all ingredients in your diffuser and use as normal.

Immune-Boosting Massage

Ingredients

2 drops Frankincense Essential Oil

2 drops Ginger Essential Oil

2 drops German Chamomile Essential Oil

1 drop Cinnamon Essential Oil

2 ounces Carrier Oil

Directions

In a small jar or container mix all ingredients until well combined. Apply topically during cold and flu season, massaging into the reflex points of the feet, or in a full-body massage.

Immune-Boosting Spray

Ingredients

    4 ounces Distilled Water

    60 drops Ginger Root Essential Oil

    20 drops Cinnamon Bark Essential Oil

Directions

Combine all ingredients in a dark colored glass spray bottle and during cold and flu season, or if there's illness in the house, spray in all rooms to stimulate the immune system.

Immune Supportive Blend

Ingredients

5 drops Melissa Essential Oil

10 drops Eucalyptus Essential Oil

10 drops Rosemary Essential Oil

15 drops Cinnamon Essential Oil

15 drops Black Pepper Essential Oil

15 drops Oregano Essential Oil

20 drops Clove Bud Essential Oil

30 drops Wild Orange Essential Oil

1:1 Coconut Oil (for external use only)

Directions

Can be used externally, internally, or aromatically.

External use: In a small glass jar, container, or roller bottle, mix all ingredients until well combined. Apply topically, massaging into the reflex points of the feet as needed, especially during cold and flu season, or whenever your immune system feels weakened.

Internal use: Double the recipe and add to an empty new 15 mL glass bottle. For immune support add 14 drops to a "00" gel capsule and take internally, once after eating every 2-3 hours. Use only three times a day for at least three days after symptoms subside.

Liver Support

Ingredients

2 drops Grapefruit Essential Oil

2 drops Clove Essential Oil

1 drop Geranium Essential Oil

1 drop Rosemary Essential Oil

1 tsp Carrier Oil

Directions

To support the liver combine all ingredients and apply topically over the region of the liver twice daily.

Mental Stimulant Bath

Ingredients

2 drops Rosemary Essential Oil

4 drops Basil Essential Oil

4 drops Lemon Essential Oil

1 Tbsp. Grapeseed Oil

Directions

To stimulate and energize your mind add all ingredients to your bathwater and stir to disperse. Inhale deeply while you soak for 20 minutes, but avoid getting water in your eyes as it may sting.

Painful Joints

Ingredients

1 cup Carrier Oil

2 drops Black Pepper Essential Oil

4 drops Cajeput Essential Oil

8 drops Eucalyptus Essential Oil

10 drops Marjoram Essential Oil

Directions

Combine all ingredients in a glass jar or dropper bottle. Place the lid on and shake vigorously to combine. Apply by massaging gently into sore muscles and joints.

Pre-Game Sports Rub

Ingredients

1 drop Lavender Essential Oil

1 drop Eucalyptus Essential Oil

2 drops Rosemary Essential Oil

4 tsps. Carrier Oil

Directions

Combine all ingredients in a glass jar or dropper bottle. Place the lid on and shake vigorously to combine. Apply by massaging gently into affected area prior to a game or exercise.

Renewing Bath

Ingredients

2 drops Juniper Berry Essential Oil

2 drops Lemon Essential Oil

4 drops Spearmint Essential Oil

4 drops Geranium Essential Oil

4 drops White Fir Essential Oil

Directions

For a refreshing bath to help you feel renewed add all ingredients to your bathwater and stir to disperse. Inhale deeply while you soak for 20 minutes, but avoid getting water in your eyes as it may sting.

Rheumatism

Ingredients

6 drops Juniper Berry Essential Oil

8 drops Lavender Essential Oil

10 drops Rosemary Essential Oil

1.5 ounces Sweet Almond Oil

Directions

In a small bowl or container mix all ingredients until well combined. To relieve rheumatism, apply topically massaging into the affected area.

Skin Toner

Ingredients

4 drops Patchouli Essential Oil

5 drops Myrrh Essential Oil

6 drops Lavender Essential Oil

8 drops Lemongrass Essential Oil

10 drops Helichrysum Essential Oil

1-ounce Carrier Oil

Directions

To smooth your skin's texture and brighten its tone combine all ingredients in a small glass bowl or container, blending well. Apply topically to the affected area up to three times daily.

Sleep Support Massage Blend

Ingredients

1 drop Cinnamon Essential Oil

4 drops Melissa Essential Oil

4 drops Marjoram Essential Oil

4 drops Pine Essential Oil

1 Tbsp. Carrier Oil

Directions

To induce a restful night's sleep combine all ingredients in a small bowl or container, blending well. Apply topically to the back of the neck, shoulders, and reflex points of the feet, inhaling the scent deeply.

Sore Muscles Massage Oil

Ingredients

15 mL Carrier Oil

3 drops Ylang Ylang Essential Oil

4 drops Bay Laurel Essential Oil

4 drops Eucalyptus Essential Oil

4 drops Rosemary Essential Oil

Directions

Combine all ingredients in a glass jar or dropper bottle. Place the lid on and shake vigorously to combine. Apply by massaging gently into sore muscles and joints.

Stress-Reducing Massage Oil

Ingredients

1 Tbsp. Carrier Oil

1 drop Lavender Essential Oil

3 drops Cinnamon Bark Essential Oil

3 drops Grapefruit Essential Oil

4 drops Fennel Essential Oil

4 drops Roman Chamomile Essential Oil

5 drops Melissa Essential Oil

Directions

In a small bowl or jar combine oils, mixing until evenly distributed. Massage the oil into the shoulders, back, and neck. Recommended for two-time use before a stressful event; 6 hours apart to help relieve anxiety.

Stress Relief

Ingredients

25 drops Wild Orange Essential Oil

20 drops Grapefruit Essential Oil

15 drops Frankincense Essential Oil

15 drops Bergamot Essential Oil

10 drops Clary Sage Essential Oil

10 drops Lemon Essential Oil

Directions

To help focus concentration combine ingredients in a bottle. Diffuse 6-7 drops as needed throughout the home or office.

Sunscreen

Ingredients

7 drops Myrrh Essential Oil

7 drops Helichrysum Essential Oil

1-ounce Carrier Oil

Instructions

For an effective sunscreen place all ingredients into a bottle and shake. Apply every two hours when you are exposed to the sun.

Sunscreen II

Ingredients

12 drops Helichrysum Essential Oil

½ cup Olive Oil

¼ cup Fractionated Coconut Oil

1 tsp. Vitamin E

2 tbsps. Zinc Oxide

2 tbsps. Shea Butter

¼ cup Beeswax

Instructions

For an effective sunscreen place all ingredients into a bottle or glass jar, blend well. Apply every two hours when you are exposed to the sun.

Varicose Veins

Ingredients

1 drop Cypress Essential Oil

1 drop Helichrysum Essential Oil

1 drop Wintergreen Essential Oil

3-4 drops Basil Essential Oil

2 Tsp Carrier Oil

Directions

To reduce the appearance of varicose veins combine all ingredients in a small bowl, blending well. Apply to the affected area, massaging gently toward the heart.

Wrinkle Salve

Ingredients

4 drops Geranium Essential Oil

3 drops Patchouli Essential Oil

3 drops Lavender Essential Oil

2 drops Frankincense Essential Oil

1-ounce Carrier Oil

Directions

To protect against or reduce the appearance of wrinkles combine all ingredients in a small glass bottle or container, blending well. Apply alongside your normal skincare regimen twice a day, morning and night.

Chapter 6:
The Ins & Outs of Essential Oils

Where do essential oils come from?

Plants and plant species naturally produce essential oils for various reasons, one being to draw pollinator insects to them, another being to repel invading organisms (bacteria, animals). A number of chemical compounds compose each plant's essential oil, and the combination of these compounds are specific to each oil, which then instills in the oil its own unique properties. Essential oils can be harnessed from all sorts of plant components, including flowers, leaves, bark, fruit, roots, and resin. For instance, Cinnamon oil is harnessed from bark, Lemon oil from the peel, and Lavender oil from Lavender flowers. Certain plants can produce a few chemical variants of the same essential oil, which are acquired from different parts of the plant. Some of these parts produce a large amount of oil, while others produce just a smidgen. The oil's quality and potency depends upon a number of factors, including the subspecies of the plant, its soil conditions, the time of year, and even the time of day you harvest it.

How are essential oils extracted?

Essential oils can be extracted from plants through various methods, including pressing, distillation, solvent, and maceration. Let's take a brief look at each:

Pressing Method

Commonly used with citrus fruit, the pressing method extracts the oil through a technique which involves pushing the fruit peels through a press. Oily fruits and plants are best suited for this technique. Orange oil, for example, is extracted from orange skins through the pressing method.

Distillation Method

This technique harkens back to the days of moonshiners, as the same sort of method used to create strong liquor can be used to extract essential oils. Using a still, boiled water, and plant materials will create steam which is then cooled by coils and condensed into a combination of water and oil. This combination doesn't mix, so the oil can then be extracted from it.

Solvent Method

Through a multi-step process, certain plant and flower oils can be extracted using alcohol and other solvents, which extort the essential oil from the plant materials.

Maceration Method

When a "carrier," fixed oil, or lard is mixed with the plant material and set out in the sun over a period of time, the carrier oil is infused with the plant's essence. Heat sources, other than the sun, are often used to speed the process. Throughout the process more plant material is added to produce a more potent oil.

How do you use essential oils?

Although some studies about the effectiveness of essential oils are conducted by small companies, or even individuals, a number of them are conducted by the food and cosmetic industries. In general, the pharmaceutical industry shows next to no interest in herbal medicine, primarily because there are few options to patent such products. As such, the product's lack of profitability results in a lack of research funding. Regardless, the historical uses of essential oils tell us what we need to know; these oils have been effectively administered for centuries. The therapeutic qualifications of essential oils can be plotted in the survival of the human race across cultures and generations.

Another reason that studies on essential oils have not resulted in much conclusive evidence as to their overall effectiveness is because definitive results are sometimes difficult to prove, as the quality of each batch of oil can vary for a number of reasons. One is that essential oils are impossible to standardize. As mentioned above, even the slightest variance in soil conditions and the time of harvesting – as well as innumerable other factors – will produce a different product quality and potency. In addition, essential oils are often obtained from various species of the same plant; Eucalyptus radiata and Eucalyptus globulus can both be used in the making of therapeutic-grade Eucalyptus oil and, as a result, they may have slightly different properties and degrees of strength or effectiveness.

Just as there are a number of methods by which to extract essential oils, there are a number of methods to administer them therapeutically. The variety of chemical compounds in each essential oil means that their benefits and applications also vary across the board. Below are a few of these methods.

Topical Administration

Direct application of many essential oils works like a sponge, as skin sops up chemicals and other things (like sunlight for instance). Topical application is best when you want to clear up an ailment on the skin's surface, or in the underlying muscle tissue. When applying topically you may either massage the oil into the skin, or simply dab on the skin for therapeutic results. You might combine the essential oil with a carrier oil for topical use in order to dilute its potency. This is safer, as the oil is so concentrated. You may support your body's defenses against rash or muscle pain in this manner, but you should always test your patient for allergies before applying. Adverse effects are produced by natural chemicals as much as synthetic ones; poison ivy, for example.

To test for allergens, place a drop or two on your patient's inner forearm. If a rash develops within 12 to 24 hours, then the patient is allergic. In addition, phototoxicity – sun exposure resulting in an exacerbated burn – may be an issue when citrus oils are applied topically. Therefore, one must proceed with caution when applying essential oils using this method.

Inhalation Therapy

Commonly known as "aromatherapy," this essential oil application is effective for inner ailments, like sore throat or cold. In a steaming bowl of distilled or sterilized water, add a few drops of essential oil and with a towel over your head, bend over the bowl and inhale. The towel captures the vapors making the technique even more effective. Essential oils can also be placed in a diffuser or potpourri throughout a room to produce somewhat diluted medicinal effects.

Ingestion

When using this method proceed with caution. Direct ingestion of essential oils must be monitored and applied in small doses that are diluted in a tablespoon or more of any carrier oil – olive oil, for example. If you are unsure of dosage amounts, make a tea with the relevant herb instead. Although the effects of this diluted use may be weaker this application is a better alternative than an overdose of essential oils.

What are the general benefits of using essential oils?

Replacement for Prescription Drugs

One practical benefit for using essential oils is their substitutive nature. Many believe that they can replace Rx drugs, which is the ultimate reason to educate yourself on their application, and to begin stockpiling your essential oil supply. Although it is our opinion that 100% pure essential oils, which carry no harmful side effects, are better to support the body and its functions, we recommend that you consult your physician before replacing your prescription, or over-the-counter medications.

One of the potential threats of economic or social collapse is the lack of resources, and primarily the inability to procure prescription drugs. As such, finding suitable alternatives should be a priority when prepping for the worst.

Their portability is also a major bonus when it comes to survival prepping. The fact that these ultra-concentrated oils take up little-to-no space makes toting them to your shelter all the easier should the need arise. Because essential oils are highly concentrated, the application used in most procedures requires only a drop or two of oil, which means that tiny bottle will be long-lasting (example 15mL bottle contains approx. 250 drops).

Cheap, but Effective Alternative

Though money may be the last thing on your mind when it comes to prepping for a survival situation (money may even be obsolete in the event of social collapse), it is worth noting that the expense of essential oils pales in comparison to prescription drugs.

No Expiration Date

Another benefit of essential oils is that they do not expire, nor do they have "proper storage" requirements. A number of medicines and medicinal products must be replaced every couple years, so this sets essential oils ahead of the pack when it comes to shelf life.

Versatility

Essential oils also offer great versatility. Aside from providing wellness benefits, essential oils can be repurposed for household and hygienic applications. For instance, if you are looking for something that might serve your dental hygiene needs in a time of crisis, Thieves Oil is your go-to essential oil. If you want to maintain your skin's health, Frankincense and Lavender will do the trick; the latter also serves as sunscreen, so you can prevent sun damage as well.

When it comes to the house or shelter you can use essential oils to deodorize, which will come in handy in a disaster scenario where things might start to smell fishy due to lack of proper utilities and care. For example, after the 2011 tsunami and the subsequent nuclear reactor meltdown in Japan, a nurse named Risa Nakahira used essential oils to deodorize and sanitize putrid public bathrooms in overpopulated evacuation facilities. As relief workers searched for survivors, often wading through debris and decay, Nakahira also deodorized their boots and masks using essential oils. The possibilities of these natural oils are endless.

They are also versatile when it comes to the range of patients they are capable of supporting. The health of everyone, from your great grandfather to your infant baby, can be fortified with the aid of essential oils in the appropriate dosage. They even come in handy when supporting livestock or pets. From teething infants to dementia in the elderly, from teenagers with acne to dogs with urinary tract infections, essential oils can serve any patient with nearly any ailment.

Conclusion

Now that you know all about what essential oils can do for you, you can start to assemble a kit of essential oils to support your anti-aging goals. Visit www.oilsclass.com to claim your free bonus video training.

The various benefits of essential oils and their properties are countless. To build your own kit, first focus on acquiring the essential oils which may bear more relevance to your aging issues or the potential health threats within your environment that may be contributing to premature aging.

ALL RIGHTS RESERVED. No part of this publication may be reproduced or transmitted in any form whatsoever, electronic, or mechanical, including photocopying, recording, or by any informational storage or retrieval system without express written, dated and signed permission from the author.

DISCLAIMER AND/OR LEGAL NOTICES: Every effort has been made to accurately represent this book and it's potential. Results vary with every individual, and your results may or may not be different from those depicted. No promises, guarantees or warranties, whether stated or implied, have been made that you will produce any specific result from this book. Your efforts are individual and unique, and may vary from those shown. Your success depends on your efforts, background and motivation.
The material in this publication is provided for educational and informational purposes only and is not intended as medical advice. The information contained in this book should not be used to diagnose or treat any illness, metabolic disorder, disease or health problem. Always consult your physician or healthcare provider before beginning any nutrition or exercise program. Use of the programs, advice, and information contained in this book is at the sole choice and risk of the reader.